Death by Medicine

Death by Medicine

by Gary Null, PhD

Martin Feldman, MD; Debora Rasio, MD;
and Carolyn Dean, MD, ND

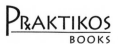

PRAKTIKOS
BOOKS

DISCLAIMER

Ideas and information in this book are based upon the experience and training of the author and the scientific information currently available. The suggestions in this book are definitely not meant to be a substitute for careful medical evaluation and treatment by a qualified, licensed health professional. The author and publisher do not recommend changing or adding medication or supplements without consulting your personal physician. They specifically disclaim any liability arising directly or indirectly from the use of this book.

Praktikos Books
P.O. Box 118
Mount Jackson, VA 22842
888.542.9467   info@praktikosbooks.com

Praktikos Books are produced in alliance with Axios Press.

Library of Congress Cataloging-in-Publication Data

Death by medicine / by Gary Null ... [et al.]. p. cm.
  Includes bibliographical references and index.
  ISBN 978-1-60766-002-6

  1. Medical errors. 2. Medical error–United States. I. Null, Gary.

R729.8.D43 2010
610–dc22

2009038210

Contents

* Iatrogenesis means "doctor-induced illness or complication."

1

Introduction

SOMETHING IS WRONG WHEN REGULATORY AGEN-
cies pretend that vitamins and nutritional
supplements are dangerous. They are not,
but some may become so if taken in renegade
doses (too high or too low), or if they are contraindicated for your condition, or when taken
with certain pharmaceuticals. So always ask
your holistic doctor before taking vitamins,
minerals, herbs, or other supplements, particularly if you are taking medications. Many in the
media, without scientific basis, denigrate the
use of supplements, yet these "vitamin critics"
ignore published statistics showing that the real
hazard is government-sanctioned medicine.

In many respects, however, these regulatory agencies act as their own critics. The government is not blind to its own deficiencies in healthcare delivery. The Institute of Medicine, a part of the United States National Academy of Sciences, states:

> Healthcare in the United States is not as safe as it should be. . . . Among the problems that commonly occur during the course of providing healthcare are adverse drug events and improper transfusions, surgical injuries and wrong-site surgery, suicides, restraint-related injuries or death, falls, burns, pressure ulcers, and mistaken patient identities [all of which exact] their cost in human lives.[1]

The Institute of Medicine even refers to "the nation's epidemic of medical errors," many of which involve adverse drug reactions (ADRs). The US Food and Drug Administration (FDA) says that "ADRs are one of the leading causes of morbidity and mortality in healthcare."[2]

Archives of Internal Medicine published "A Special Article" by Curt D. Furberg, MD, PhD, et al., called "The FDA and Drug Safety: A Proposal for Sweeping Changes." The section "Problems with the Current System" begins: "We see eight major problems with the current system of assessment and assurance of drug safety at the FDA." The first of these says that the initial review for approval often fails to detect serious ADRs: "A study by the US General Accountability Office (GAO) concluded that 51% of all approved drugs had at least one serious ADR that was not recognized during the approval process."[3]

The irony is that safer (and less expensive) preventive alternatives are often attacked or strategically ridiculed by regulatory powers, even—or perhaps especially—when proven effective. This condescending stance toward alternatives may be fueled by their relative lack of side effects in a competitive marketplace.

Until recently, health researchers could cite only isolated statistics to make their case about the dangers of conventional medicine. No one had ever analyzed and compiled all the published literature dealing with injuries and deaths caused by government-protected medicine.

A group of researchers meticulously reviewed the statistical evidence, and their findings, included in this book, are absolutely shocking. In *Death by Medicine*, we will present compelling evidence that today's healthcare system frequently causes more harm than good.

This fully referenced book reveals a number of startling facts:

- The number of people having in-hospital, adverse reactions to prescribed drugs annually: approximately 2.2 million
- The number of unnecessary and/or inappropriate antibiotics prescribed annually: approximately 45 million per year[4, 5]
- The number of unnecessary medical and surgical procedures performed each year: 7.5 million
- The number of people unnecessarily hospitalized each year: 8.9 million

The most stunning statistic, however, is that the total number of deaths caused by conventional medicine is nearly 800,000 per year. It is now evident that the American medical system is the leading cause of death and injury in the US. By contrast, the number of deaths attributable to heart disease in 2005, the most recent year for which final data is available, is 652,091, while the number of deaths attributable to cancer is 559,312.[6] "It is estimated that . . . 565,650 men and women will die of cancer of all sites in 2008," according to the National Cancer Institute, a projected increase of 6,338 cancer deaths.[7]

We decided to publish *Death by Medicine* to call attention to the failure of the American medical system. By exposing these gruesome statistics in painstaking detail, we provide a basis for competent and compassionate medical professionals, such as the courageous Dr. David Graham, to recognize the inadequacies of today's system and at least attempt to institute meaningful reforms.

On November 18, 2004, David J. Graham, MD, MPH, Associate Director for Science and Medicine in the FDA's Office of Drug Safety, testified before the US Senate. Dr. Graham graduated from the Johns Hopkins University School of Medicine, and trained in Internal Medicine at Yale and in adult Neurology at the University of Pennsylvania. After this, he completed a three-year fellowship in pharmaco-epidemiology and a Masters in Public Health at Johns Hopkins, with a concentration in epidemiology and biostatistics.[8] His education and extensive experience qualify him to offer an expert opinion on pharmaceutical drugs.

Dr. Graham, who had spent twenty years working at the FDA, told the Senate:

> During my career, I believe I have made a real difference for the cause of patient safety. My research and efforts within FDA led to the withdrawal from the US market of Omniflox, an antibiotic that caused hemolytic anemia; Rezulin, a diabetes drug that caused acute liver failure; Fen-Phen and Redux, weight loss drugs that caused heart valve injury; and PPA (phenylpropanolamine), an over-the-counter decongestant and weight

loss product that caused hemorrhagic stroke in young women.

My research also led to the withdrawal from outpatient use of Trovan, an antibiotic that caused acute liver failure and death. I also contributed to the team effort that led to the withdrawal of Lotronex, a drug for irritable bowel syndrome that causes ischemic colitis; Baycol, a cholesterol-lowering drug that caused severe muscle injury, kidney failure and death; Seldane, an antihistamine that caused heart arrhythmias and death; and Propulsid, a drug for night-time heartburn that caused heart arrhythmias and death. . . .

I have done extensive work concerning the issue of pregnancy exposure to Accutane, a drug that is used to treat acne but can cause birth defects in some children who are exposed *in utero* if their mothers take the drug during the first trimester. During my career, I have recommended the market withdrawal of twelve drugs. Only two of these remain on the market today—Accutane and Arava, a drug for the treatment of rheumatoid arthritis that I and a co-worker believe causes an unacceptably high risk of acute liver failure and death.[9]

The *Los Angeles Times* reported that witnesses told the Senate panel that

Merck & Co. and the Food and Drug Administration knew before the agency approved the company's Vioxx® painkiller in 1999 that the drug could have serious adverse effects on the heart. . . . But the FDA gave its approval without resolving the concerns, and Vioxx® was aggressively marketed to point up its pain relief qualities, not its risks.[10]

Testifying about Merck's Vioxx®, Dr. Graham states:

Today . . . you, we, are faced with what may be the single greatest drug safety catastrophe in the history of this country or the history of the world. We are talking about a catastrophe that I strongly believe could have, should have, been largely or completely avoided. But it wasn't, and over 100,000 Americans have paid dearly for this failure. In my opinion, the FDA has let the American people down, and sadly, betrayed a public trust.[11]

In the same way the FDA attempts to quash vitamins, they allegedly attempted to suppress scientific research, presumably to keep Vioxx® and other drugs afloat, according to Dr. Graham. "Not only did the FDA ignore known risks from Vioxx® and related drugs but . . . it tried to prevent Graham and others from publicizing their own research that proved the extent of these risks."[12]

When it comes to new medications, Attorney Blake Bailey observes:

The FDA . . . uses the studies of the companies who stand to gain billions of dollars and are under intense pressure to beat a competing company to make it to the market with a similar product. Many of the scientists and medical doctors go to work for these companies after a tenure with FDA.[13]

Dr. Graham made it clear in his testimony that, throughout his career, he had only worked for the FDA, not for any companies.

Committee Chairman Charles E. Grassley (R–Iowa) said he was concerned that the FDA "has a relationship with drug companies that is too cozy."[14]

Sen. Jeff Bingaman (D–New Mexico) said the problem was within the FDA's own culture: "The culture within the FDA, being one where the pharmaceutical industry, which the FDA is supposed to regulate, is seen by the FDA as its client instead.[15]

In Graham's view, the drug safety problems began in 1992 with the passage of a law aimed at getting lifesaving drugs onto the market faster. To speed up approvals, the law forced pharmaceutical companies to foot most of the bill for the review process. That left the FDA "captured by industry," says Graham. "He who pays the piper calls the tune."[16]

Edward J. Markey (D–Massachusetts) noted that a 2006 survey conducted by the Union of Concerned Scientists reported that 18.4% of FDA scientists surveyed reported that they had been asked to inappropriately exclude or alter technical information or their conclusions in an FDA scientific document.[17]

The American Society of Health-System Pharmacists reports that Graham testified "in February [2007] that, had it not been for the protection of Sen. Charles Grassley (R–Iowa), FDA would have fired him for publicly speaking out about his concerns about Vioxx® and other drugs."[18]

Dr. Graham says, "You need to weed the garden patch of drugs that aren't doing what they're supposed to do. The FDA has not been very good about that; it likes to cultivate all these weeds."[19] Dr. Graham "named five other drugs whose safety is suspect, and noted that 'the FDA as currently configured is incapable of protecting America against another Vioxx®.'"[20]

Many media sources present at the hearing, such as the *Los Angeles Times* and *Medscape Medical News*,[21] report that Graham then added, "We are virtually defenseless,"[22] but this sentence does not appear in the final transcript and may have been stricken from the record. One report begins, "The American public is 'virtually defenseless' if another medication such as Vioxx® proves to be unsafe after it is approved for sale, a government drug safety reviewer told a congressional committee."[23]

Yet the FDA crusades to prevent us from taking dandelion root.

Natural medicine is under siege, as pharmaceutical company lobbyists urge lawmakers to deprive Americans of the benefits of dietary supplements and bioidentical hormones. Drug-company front groups have launched slanderous media campaigns to discredit the value of healthy lifestyles. The FDA continues to interfere with those who offer natural products that compete with prescription drugs.

These attacks against natural medicine obscure a lethal problem that until now was buried in thousands of pages of scientific text. In response to these baseless challenges to natural medicine, here is an independent review of the quality of "government-approved" medicine. To support the bold claim that conventional medicine is America's number one killer, every count in this indictment of US medicine is validated by published, peer-reviewed scientific studies. The startling findings from this meticulous study indicate that conventional medicine is the leading cause of death in the United States.

What you are about to read is a stunning compilation of facts that documents that those who seek to abolish consumer access to natural therapies are misleading the public. Nearly 800,000 Americans die each year at the hands of government-sanctioned medicine, while the FDA and other government agencies pretend to protect the public by harassing those who offer safe alternatives.

A definitive review of medical peer-reviewed journals and government health statistics shows that American medicine frequently causes more harm than good.

Each year at least 2.2 million US hospital patients experience adverse drug reactions (ADRs) to prescribed medications.[24] The FDA acknowledges that, compared with data from the Institutes of Medicine, studies

> conducted on hospitalized patient populations have placed much higher estimates on the overall incidence of serious ADRs. These studies estimate that 6.7% of hospitalized patients have a serious adverse drug reaction with a fatality rate of 0.32%.[25]

> If these estimates are correct, then there are more than 2,216,000 serious ADRs in hospitalized patients, causing over 106,000 deaths annually. . . . These statistics do not include the number of ADRs that occur in ambulatory settings. Also, it is estimated that over 350,000 ADRs occur in US nursing homes each year.[26] The exact number of ADRs is not certain and is limited by methodological considerations. However, whatever the

true number is, ADRs represent a significant public health problem that is, for the most part, preventable.[27]

In 1995, Dr. Richard Besser of the federal Centers for Disease Control and Prevention (CDC) estimated the number of unnecessary antibiotics prescribed annually for viral infections to be 20 million; in 2003, Dr. Besser spoke in terms of tens of millions of unnecessary antibiotics prescribed annually.[28, 29]

In 2005, Dr. Philip Tierno, director of clinical microbiology and immunology at New York University Medical Center said that each year "about 90 million antibiotic prescriptions are written and about half of those are either unnecessary or inappropriate, which is the leading cause of antibiotic resistance in America."[30]

In October 2008, Dr. Lauri Hicks, medical director of the CDC's Get Smart: Know When Antibiotics Work program, warns: "Antibiotic overuse is a serious problem and a threat to everyone's health." The CDC reports, "Upper respiratory tract infections [are] usually caused by viruses [and] can't be cured with antibiotics. Yet each year, healthcare providers in the US prescribe tens of millions of antibiotics for viral infections." Dr. Hicks explains, "Taking antibiotics when you don't need them or not as prescribed increases your risk of getting an infection later that resists antibiotic treatment."[31]

The CDC announced that to bring attention to this increasing problem, they initiated a Get Smart About Antibiotics Week in 2008, a campaign to educate the public[32] and, by implication, to sensitize physicians to the danger of over-prescribing, a practice that has been building with impunity for many years, but which can no longer be readily tolerated.

Approximately 7.5 million unnecessary medical and surgical procedures are performed annually in the US,[33, 34] while approximately 8.9 million Americans are hospitalized unnecessarily.[35–38] The Institute of Medicine estimates that nearly 100,000 patients die in hospitals each year due to medical errors. This is three times the number who die on the highways.[39]

Deaths from nosocomial infections—that is, infections that are a result of treatment in a hospital or a healthcare service unit, appearing 48 hours or more after hospital admission or within 30 days after discharge—rose from 88,000 in 1997[40, 41] to 99,000 per year in 2002.[42] According to the CDC, in American hospitals alone, healthcare-associated infections (HAIs) account for an estimated 1.7 million infections and 99,000 associated deaths each year."[43] There were

- 33,269 HAIs among newborns in high-risk nurseries,
- 19,059 among newborns in well-baby nurseries,
- 417,946 among adults and children in ICUs, and
- 1,266,851 among adults and children outside of ICUs.

Of the 99,000 associated deaths,

- 35,967 were for pneumonia,
- 30,665 for bloodstream infections,
- 13,088 for urinary tract infections,
- 8,205 for surgical site infections, and
- 11,062 for infections of other sites.[44]

As shown in Table 1, the estimated total number of iatrogenic deaths—that is, deaths induced inadvertently by a physician or surgeon or by medical treatment or diagnostic procedures—in the US annually is at least 794,936. It is evident that the American medical system is itself the leading cause of death and injury in the US. By comparison, approximately 652,091 Americans died of heart disease in 2005, while 559,312 died of cancer.[45]

The mortality costs alone exceed $282 billion a year. "Healthcare costs in the United States are growing at an unsustainable rate," according to Senator Ron Wyden, who serves on the Senate's Finance Committee, Subcommittee on Healthcare.[46]

The National Coalition on Healthcare reports that annual healthcare spending in the US has been increasing two to five times the rate of inflation since 2000.[47] In 2006, Americans spent more than $2.2 trillion on healthcare.[48] Total healthcare spending was $2.4 trillion in both 2007 and 2008, or $7,900 per person, which represented 17 percent of the gross domestic product

Table 1: Estimated Annual Mortality and Cost of Medical Intervention

Condition	Deaths	Cost	Author
Hospital Adverse Drug Reactions	106,000+	$12 billion+	Lazarou,[49] Suh,[50] FDA[51]
Hospital Medical Errors	98,000	$2 billion	IOM,[52][53][54]
Hospital Bedsores	115,000	$55 billion	Xakellis,[55] Barczak,[56]
Hospital Infections	99,000	$5 billion+	CDC,[57] Weinstein,[58] MMWR[59]
Nursing Homes/Malnutrition	108,800	-----------	Coalition for Nursing Home Reform[60]
Outpatient Adverse Drug Reactions	199,000	77 billion	Starfield,[61][62] Weingart[63]
Unnecessary Surgical Procedures	37,136	$122 billion	HCUP[64][65]
Surgery-Related	32,000	$9 billion	AHRQ[66]
Total	**794,936+**	**$282 billion +**	

(GDP).[67] That's about 4.3 times the amount spent on national defense.[68] The total was projected to reach $3.1 trillion in 2012.[69]

The National Coalition on Healthcare further states:

> It is estimated that we have spent as a nation nearly 16 trillion dollars on healthcare since 2000, but this expenditure has not resulted in demonstrably better quality of care or better patient satisfaction compared to other nations.[70]

Jason Lazarou, MSc, estimated 106,000 annual drug errors in his groundbreaking 1998 report in the *Journal of the American Medical Association*;[71] the Institute of Medicine estimated 98,000 annual medical errors. But if we use Dr. Lucian L. Leape's 1997 medical and drug error rate of 3 million[72] multiplied by the 14% fatality rate he used in 1994,[73] we find that the number of deaths would be increased by 216,000, for a total of 1,010,936 deaths annually, as shown in Table 2 (next page).

Table 2: Estimated Annual Mortality and Cost of Medical Intervention

Condition	Deaths	Cost	Reference
Hospital ADR/med error	420,000	$200 billion	Leape [74]
Hospital Bedsores	115,000	$55 billion	Xakellis,[75] Barczak[76]
Hospital Infection	99,000	$5 billion+	CDC,[77] Weinstein[78] MMWR[79]
Nursing Home/Malnutrition	108,800	----------	Coalition for Nursing Home Reform[80]
Outpatients	199,000	$77 billion	Starfield,[81, 82] Weingart[83]
Unnecessary Procedures	37,136	$122 billion	HCUP[84]
Surgery-Related	32,000	$9 billion	AHRQ[85]
Total	**1,010,936**	**$468 billion +**	

"In the past, medicine was 'simple, relatively safe, and ineffective'. . . but today medicine is complicated . . . which has made it less safe, and it is still ineffective," according to Dr. Leape.[86] Emergency medicine helps many.

Unnecessary medical events, including pointless hospitalization, are important in our analysis. These events are among the most lamentable in all of medicine. They are usually preventable. Any invasive inappropriate medical procedure puts a patient at risk for an iatrogenic cascade of injuries, possibly death. Unfortunately, cause and effect go unmonitored. "At least 150 times [in the seven years between 1996 and 2003], surgeons in American hospitals have operated on the wrong arm, leg, eye or other body part."

Do not imagine that hospitals viewed as role models for research and fine clinical care are perfect. Memorial Sloan–Kettering Cancer Center in New York City "advertises that it delivers the best cancer care anywhere. But in 1995, its chief neurosurgeon operated on the wrong side of a patient's brain in part because of a mix-up in X-rays. . . . Lapses in basic quality checks and ordinary standards of patient care led to most of the mishaps."[87]

The figures on unnecessary events represent people who are thrust into a dangerous health-care system. Each of these 16.4 million lives is being affected in ways that could have fatal consequences. Simply entering a hospital could result in the following:

- In 16.4 million people, a 2.1% chance (affecting 344,400) of a serious adverse drug reaction[88]
- In 16.4 million people, a 5–6% chance (affecting 902,000) of acquiring a noso-comial infection[89]
- In 16.4 million people, a 4–36% chance (affecting between 656,000 and 5.9 million) of having an iatrogenic injury (medical error or adverse drug reactions)[90]
- In 16.4 million people, a 17% chance (affecting 2.8 million) of a procedure error[91]

These statistics represent a one-year time span. Working with the most conservative figures from our statistics, we project the following ten-year death rates (Table 3):

Table 3: Estimated 10-Year Death Rates from Medical Intervention

Condition	10YearDeaths	Reference
Hospital Adverse Drug Reaction	1.06 million +	Lazarou[92]
Hospital Medical Error	0.98 million	IOM[93, 94, 95]
Hospital Bedsores	1.15 million	Xakellis,[96] Barczak[97]
Hospital Infection	0.99 million	CDC,[98] Weinstein,[99] MMWR[100]
Nursing Home/Malnutrition	1.09 million	Coalition for Nursing Home Reform[101]
Outpatients	1.99 million	Starfield,[102, 103] Weingart[104]
Unnecessary Procedures	371,360	HCUP[105]
Surgery-related	320,000	AHRQ[106]
Total	**7,951,360 +**	

Our estimated ten-year total of 7.95 million iatrogenic deaths is more than all the casualties from all the wars fought by the US throughout its entire history. Our projected figures for unnecessary medical events occurring over a ten-year period are also striking. The figures in Table 4 show that an estimated 164 million people—more than half of the total US population—receive unneeded medical treatment over the course of a decade.

Table 4: Estimated Ten-Year Unnecessary Medical Events

Unnecessary Events	10-year Number	Iatrogenic Events
Hospitalization	89 million[107–110]	17 million
Procedures	75 million[111]	15 million
Total	**164 million**	**32 million**

2

Medically Induced Death: The Equivalent of Six Jumbo Jets Falling Out of the Sky Each Day

NEVER BEFORE HAVE COMPLETE STATISTICS ON the multiple causes of iatrogenesis been combined in one book. Medical science amasses tens of thousands of papers annually, each representing a tiny fragment of the whole picture. To look at only one piece and try to understand the benefits and risks is like standing an inch away from an elephant and trying to describe everything about it. You have to step back to see the big picture, as we have done here. Each specialty, each division of medicine, keeps its own records and data on morbidity and mortality. We have now completed the painstaking work of reviewing thousands of studies and putting the pieces of the puzzle together.

Is American Medicine Working?

US healthcare spending reached $1.6 trillion in 2003, representing 14% of the nation's gross national product.[112] When spending rose to $2.4 trillion per year in 2007, it would represent 17% of the gross domestic product.[113] Considering this enormous expenditure, which occurred in 2008 as well, we should have the best medicine in the world. We should be preventing and reversing disease, and doing minimal harm. Careful and objective review, however, shows we are doing the opposite. Because of the extraordinarily narrow, technologically driven context in which contemporary medicine examines the human condition, we are completely missing the larger picture.

Medicine is not taking into consideration the following critically important aspects of a healthy human organism:

- stress, and how it adversely affects the immune system and life processes;
- insufficient exercise;
- excessive calorie intake;
- highly processed and denatured foods, grown in denatured and chemically damaged soil; and
- exposure to tens of thousands of environmental toxins.

Instead of minimizing these disease-causing factors, we cause more illness through medical technology, diagnostic testing, overuse of medical and surgical procedures, and overuse of pharmaceutical drugs. The huge disservice of this therapeutic strategy is the result of little effort or money being spent on preventing disease, as evidenced by efforts to curtail use of effective vitamins and supplements. The recent article, "US Spends $700 Billion on Unnecessary Medical Tests," which appears on the

Healthcare Economist website, reflects the state of our techno-med nation:

> Peter Orszag, director of the Congressional Budget Office, estimates that 5 percent of the nation's gross domestic product—$700 billion per year—goes to tests and procedures that do not actually improve health outcomes. . . . The unreasonably high cost of healthcare in the United States is a deeply entrenched problem that must be attacked at its root." This quotation comes from a Progressive Policy Institute (PPI) report. There is little doubt that much of healthcare is unnecessary or at least is not worthwhile in the cost-benefit sense.[114]

Moreover,

> Some medical experts say the American devotion to the newest, most expensive technology is an important reason that the United States spends much more on healthcare than other

industrialized nations. . . without providing better care. . . . [A] Rand Corporation study estimated that one-third or more of the care that patients in this country receive could be of little value. If that is so, hundreds of billions of dollars each year are being wasted on superfluous treatments.

[There is] a much larger trend in American medicine. . . . A faith in innovation, often driven by [quick] financial incentives, encourages American doctors and hospitals to adopt new technologies even without proof that they work better than older techniques. . . . The problem is not that newer treatments never work. It is that once they become available, [too often prematurely,] they are often used indiscriminately, in the absence of studies to determine which patients they will benefit. . . . And sometimes, the new technologies prove harmful. . . . [Some] doctors in private practice who own their [CT] scanners, use

> the tests aggressively . . . [as if it were]
> a new toy in the office[115]

—endangering asymptomatic patients for whom the scan may be inappropriate.

Health Insurance

To determine whether American medicine is working, we also need to know if enough people have access to the American healthcare system. The National Coalition on Healthcare reports, "Nearly 46 million Americans, or 18 percent of the population under the age of 65, were without health insurance in 2007, the latest government data available."[116] As of September 2007, one out of three Americans were uninsured. [117, 118] This number is apt to rise sharply for 2008 and 2009 because so many Americans are losing their jobs in the recession.

> The number of uninsured children in 2007 was 8.1 million—or 10.7 percent of all children in the US. . . . The large majority of the uninsured (80 percent) are native or naturalized citizens. . . .

The number of uninsured rose 2.2 million between 2005 and 2006 and has increased by almost 8 million people since 2000. . . .

A study found that 29 percent of people who had health insurance were "underinsured" with coverage so meager they often postponed medical care because of costs. Nearly 50 percent overall, and 43 percent of people with health coverage, said they were "somewhat" to "completely" unprepared to cope with a costly medical emergency over the coming year.[119]

The National Coalition on Healthcare advises,

Getting everyone covered will save lives and money. The impacts of going uninsured are clear and severe. Many uninsured individuals postpone needed medical care which results in increased mortality and billions of dollars lost in productivity and increased expenses to the healthcare system.[120]

The Los Angeles Times almost waxes poetic about healthcare insurance as journalist Ricardo Alonso-Zaldivar observes, "Some people marry for love, some for companionship, and others for status or money. Now comes another reason to get hitched: health insurance."[121]

> A poll of 2,003 adults released on April 27, 2008 (on the cusp of our economic recession) by the Kaiser Family Foundation found that "7% of Americans said they or someone in their household decided to marry in the last year so they could get healthcare benefits via their spouse." Not surprisingly, "Those who cited health insurance as a factor in deciding to marry tended to have modest incomes. About 6 in 10 were in households making less than $50,000 a year, said Mollyann Brodie, who directs Kaiser's opinion research." What surprised researchers was that such costs had become a factor in marriage decisions. "We should have asked about divorce," said Drew

E. Altman, president of the Kaiser Family Foundation, "joking."[122]

The Institute of Medicine found that the 41 million Americans with no health insurance have consistently worse clinical outcomes than those who are insured, and are at increased risk for dying prematurely.[123]

Compounding the problem is the issue of insurance fraud. When doctors bill for services they do not render, advise unnecessary tests, or screen everyone for a rare condition, they are committing insurance fraud. The US GAO estimated that $12 billion was lost to fraudulent or unnecessary claims in 1998, and reclaimed $480 million in judgments in that year. In 2001, the federal government won or negotiated more than $1.7 billion in judgments, settlements, and administrative impositions in healthcare fraud cases and proceedings.[124]

Underreporting of Iatrogenic Events

As little as 5% and no more than 20% of iatrogenic events are ever reported.[125, 126–129] This implies that if medical errors were completely and accurately reported, we would have an annual iatrogenic death toll much higher than 794,936. In 1994, Leape said his figure of 180,000 medical mistakes resulting in death annually was equivalent to three jumbo jet crashes every two days.[130] Our considerably higher figure is equivalent to six jumbo jets falling out of the sky each day.

What we must deduce from this report is that medicine is in need of complete and total reform—from the curriculum in medical schools to protecting patients from excessive medical intervention. It is obvious that we cannot change anything if we are not honest about what needs to be changed. This report simply shows the degree to which change is required.

We are fully aware of what stands in the way of change: powerful pharmaceutical and medical technology companies, along with other powerful groups with enormous vested interests in the business of medicine. They fund medical research, support medical schools and hospitals, and advertise in medical journals. With deep pockets, they entice scientists and academics to support their efforts. Such funding can sway the balance of opinion from professional caution to uncritical acceptance of new therapies and drugs. You have only to look at the people who make up the hospital, medical, and government health advisory boards to see conflicts of interest.

For example, a 2003 study found that nearly half of medical school faculty who serve on institutional review boards (IRBs) to advise on clinical trial research also serve as consultants to the pharmaceutical industry.[131] The study authors were concerned that such representation could cause potential conflicts of interest. In a news release, Dr. Erik Campbell, the lead author, wrote, "Our previous research with faculty has shown us that ties to industry can affect scientific behavior, leading to such things as trade secrecy and delays in publishing research. It's possible that similar relationships with companies could affect IRB members' activities and attitudes."[132] The public is mostly unaware of these interlocking interests. (For more on this, see chapter 8, "Medical Ethics and Conflict of Interest in Scientific Medicine.")

Government medical advisors play a role in adequate reporting of iatrogenic events. The FDA announced in March 2007:

> Expert advisers to the government who receive money from a drug or device maker would be barred for the first time from voting on whether to approve that company's products under new rules . . . for the FDA's powerful advisory committees. Indeed, such doctors who receive more than $50,000 from a company or a competitor whose product is being discussed would no longer be allowed to serve on the committees, though those who receive less than that amount in the prior year can join a committee and participate in its discussions. A "significant number" of

the agency's present advisers would be affected by the new policy, said the FDA acting deputy commissioner, Randall W. Lutter, though he would not say how many.[133]

The First Study of Iatrogenesis

Dr. Lucian L. Leape opened medicine's Pandora's box in his 1994 paper, "Error in Medicine," which appeared in the *Journal of the American Medical Association (JAMA)*.[134] He noted that Schimmel reported in 1964 that 20% of hospital patients suffered iatrogenic injury, with a 20% fatality rate. In 1981, Steel reported that 36% of hospitalized patients experienced iatrogenesis, with a 25% fatality rate, and adverse drug reactions were involved in 50% of the injuries. In 1991, Bedell reported that 64% of acute heart attacks in one hospital were preventable and were mostly due to adverse drug reactions.

Leape focused on the Harvard Medical Practice Study published in 1991,[135] which found a 4% iatrogenic injury rate for patients, with a 14% fatality rate, in 1984 in New York State.

From the 98,609 patients injured and the 14% fatality rate, he estimated that in the entire US, 180,000 people die each year partly as a result of iatrogenic injury.

Why Leape chose to use the much lower figure of 4% injury for his analysis remains in question. Using instead the average of the rates found in the three studies he cites (36%, 20%, and 4%) would have produced a 20% medical error rate. The number of iatrogenic deaths using an average rate of injury and his 14% fatality rate would be 1,189,576.

Leape acknowledged that the literature on medical errors is sparse and represents only the tip of the iceberg, noting that when errors are specifically sought out, reported rates are "distressingly high." He cited several autopsy studies with rates as high as 35–40% of missed diagnoses causing death. He also noted that an intensive care unit reported an average of 1.7 errors per day per patient, and 29% of those errors were potentially serious or fatal.

Leape calculated the error rate in the intensive care unit study. First, he found that each patient had an average of 178 "activities" (staff/procedure/medical interactions) a day, of which 1.7 were errors, which means a 1% failure rate. This may not seem like much, but Leape cited industry standards showing that in aviation, a 0.1% failure rate would mean two unsafe plane landings per day at Chicago's O'Hare International Airport; in the US Postal Service, a 0.1% failure rate would mean 16,000 pieces of lost mail every hour; and in the banking industry, a 0.1% failure rate would mean 32,000 bank checks deducted from the wrong bank account.

At the same time, Leape acknowledged the lack of reporting of medical errors. Medical errors occur in thousands of different locations and are perceived as isolated and unusual events. But the most important reason that the problem of medical errors is unrecognized and growing, according to Leape, is that doctors and nurses are unequipped to deal with human error because of the culture of medical training and practice.

Doctors are taught that mistakes are unacceptable. Medical mistakes are therefore viewed as a failure of character and any error equals negligence. No one is taught what to do when medical errors do occur. Leape cites McIntyre and Popper, who said the "infallibility model" of medicine leads to intellectual dishonesty with a need to cover up mistakes rather than admit them.

There are no Grand Rounds on medical errors, no sharing of failures among doctors, and no one to support them emotionally when their error harms a patient. Leape hoped his paper would encourage medical practitioners "to fundamentally change the way they think about errors and why they occur." It has been almost a decade since this groundbreaking work, but the mistakes continue to soar.

In 1995, a *JAMA* report noted, "Over a million patients are injured in US hospitals each year, and approximately 280,000 die annually as a result of these injuries. Therefore, the iatrogenic death rate dwarfs the annual automobile accident mortality rate of 45,000 and accounts for more deaths than all other accidents combined."[136]

At a 1997 press conference, Leape released a nationwide poll on patient iatrogenesis conducted by the National Patient Safety Foundation (NPSF), which is sponsored by the American Medical Association (AMA). Leape is a founding member of NPSF. The survey found that more than 100 million Americans have been affected directly or indirectly by a medical mistake. Forty-two percent were affected directly and 84% personally knew of someone who had experienced a medical mistake.[137]

At this press conference, Leape updated his 1994 statistics, noting that as of 1997, medical errors in inpatient hospital settings nationwide could be as high as 3 million and could cost as much as $200 billion. Leape used a 14% fatality rate to determine a medical error death rate of 180,000 in 1994.[138] In 1997, using Leape's base number of 3 million errors, the annual death rate could be as high as 420,000 for hospital inpatients alone.

Only a Fraction of Medical Errors Are Reported

> If the medical system were a bank, you wouldn't deposit your money here, because there would be an error every one-in-two to one-in-three times you made a transaction.
>
> STEPHEN PERSELL, MD, Northwestern University's Feinberg School of Medicine[139]

In 1994, Leape said he was well aware that medical errors were not being reported.[140] A study conducted in two obstetrical units in the UK found that only about one quarter of adverse incidents were ever reported, to protect staff, preserve reputations, or for fear of reprisals, including lawsuits.[141]

An analysis by Wald and Shojania found that only 1.5% of all adverse events result in an incident report, and only 6% of adverse drug events are identified properly. The authors learned that the American College of Surgeons estimates that surgical incident reports routinely capture only 5–30% of adverse events. In one study, only 20% of surgical complications resulted in discussion at morbidity and mortality rounds.[142]

From these studies, it appears that all the statistics gathered on medical errors may substantially underestimate the number of adverse drug and medical therapy incidents. They also suggest that our statistics concerning mortality resulting from medical errors may be in fact conservative figures.

An article in *Psychiatric Times* (April 2000) outlines the stakes involved in reporting medical errors.[143] The authors found that the public is fearful of suffering a fatal medical error, and doctors are afraid they will be sued if they report an error. This brings up the obvious question: who is reporting medical errors? Usually it is the patient or the patient's surviving family. If no one notices the error, it is never reported.

Janet Heinrich, an associate director at the US General Accountability Office responsible for health financing and public health issues, testified before a House subcommittee hearing on medical errors that "the full magnitude of their threat to the American public is unknown" and "gathering valid and useful information about adverse events is extremely difficult." She acknowledged that the fear of being blamed, and the potential for legal liability, played key roles in the underreporting of errors.

The *Psychiatric Times* noted that the AMA strongly opposes mandatory reporting of medical errors.[144] If doctors are not reporting, what about nurses? A survey of nurses found that they also fail to report medical mistakes for fear of retaliation.[145]

No Improvement in Error Reporting

A 2003 survey is all the more distressing because there seems to be no improvement in error reporting, even with all the attention given to this topic. Dr. Dorothea Wild surveyed medical residents at a community hospital in Connecticut and found that only half were aware that the hospital had a medical error-reporting system, and that the vast majority did not use it at all. Dr. Wild says this does not bode well for the future. If doctors do not learn error reporting in their training, they will never use it. Wild adds that error reporting is the first step in locating the gaps in the medical system and fixing them.[146]

In their article, "Underreporting of Medical Errors Affecting Children Is a Significant Problem, Particularly among Physicians," the Agency for Healthcare Research and Quality (AHRQ) reports that a study in 2004 published in the journal *Pediatrics* discovered that most medical errors made by nurses and physicians treating children are never reported.[147, 148]

On February 17, 2008, Indiana University School of Medicine aired a revealing radio interview with Lauris Kaldjian, MD, PhD, of the Dept. of Internal Medicine and Program in Biomedical Ethics at the University of Iowa's Roy J. and Lucille A. Carver College of Medicine. The program was called, "Doctors Don't Report Medical Errors." A question is posed:

> Let's say you're a doctor—a heart surgeon. And you make a mistake. Maybe you prescribe the wrong medicine.

Maybe you cut something you're not supposed to. And it might not be a big deal. But then again, it might. The question is: do you admit your mistake and report it to the higher ups?

Lauris Kaldjian directs the bioethics program at the University of Iowa. According to his recent study, the answer to that question is probably no. Most doctors he surveyed agree in theory that's it's a good thing to report medical errors. But few actually do it.[149]

Dr. Kaldjian's report on medical errors appears in the January 14, 2008, issue of the *Archives of Internal Medicine*.

Medical Errors a Global Issue

A five-country survey published in the *Journal of Health Affairs* found that 18–28% of people who were recently ill had suffered from a medical or drug error in the previous two years. The study surveyed 750 recently ill adults. The breakdown by country showed the percentages of those suffering a medical or drug error were 18% in Britain, 23% in Australia and in New Zealand, 25% in Canada, and 28% in the US.[150]

Public Suggestions on Iatrogenesis

In a telephone survey, 1,207 adults ranked the effectiveness of the following measures in reducing preventable medical errors that result in serious harm.[151] Following each measure is the percentage of respondents who ranked the measure as "very effective."

- Giving doctors more time to spend with patients (78%)
- Requiring hospitals to develop systems to avoid medical errors (74%)
- Better training of health professionals (73%)
- Using only doctors specially trained in intensive care medicine on intensive care units (73%)
- Requiring hospitals to report all serious medical errors to a state agency (71%)

- Increasing the number of hospital nurses (69%)
- Reducing the work hours of doctors in training to avoid fatigue (66%)
- Encouraging hospitals to voluntarily report serious medical errors to a state agency (62%)

Various initiatives are under way to address these problems. The Patient Safety and Quality Improvement Act of 2005[152] "was enacted in response to growing concern about patient safety in the United States. . . . The goal of the Act is to improve patient safety by encouraging voluntary and confidential reporting of events that adversely affect patients."[153] The success of this legislation will depend in large part upon the willingness of healthcare providers to reveal errors of colleagues, as well as their own in a challenging medical environment that reveres the concept of accuracy.

A new specialty in modern medicine that is developing in part from the focus on the need for improved quality of hospital care is Hospital Medicine. It trains physicians as "hospitalists" to devote themselves to the safety of hospital patients. These would be the doctors referred to above who are "specially trained in intensive care medicine on intensive care units." These would also be the physicians who are there to relieve doctors in training, which would allow doctors' shifts to be reduced in order to combat fatigue and reduce errors. In 2009, The American Board of Hospital Medicine (ABHM), was founded as the first board of certification for Hospital Medicine in North America. The specialized training of "hospitalists" and the increase in their future numbers may enable them to spend more time with patients, which appears to be a priority with the public. There are also campaigns to increase the number of hospital nurses and to educate them regarding hospital errors.

3

Problems with Drugs

PRESCRIPTION DRUGS CONSTITUTE THE MAJOR treatment modality of scientific medicine. With the discovery of the "germ theory," medical scientists convinced the public that infectious organisms were the cause of illness. Finding the "cure" for these infections proved much harder than anyone imagined. From the beginning, chemical drugs promised much more than they delivered. But far beyond not working, the drugs also caused incalculable side effects. The drugs themselves, even when properly prescribed, have side effects that can be fatal, as Lazarou's study[154] showed. But human error can make the situation even worse.

On December 10, 2007, the headline read: "The Quaid Twins 'Fighting for Their Lives': Dennis and Kimberly Quaid Keep Vigil as Their Newborns Struggle to Survive a Devastating Hospital Error that Resulted in an Overdose of Blood Thinner":

> The twins were hospitalized at Cedars-Sinai [Medical Center in L.A.] due to staph infections. . . . At the hospital on Nov. 18, [2007,] they were allegedly among three patients given 1,000 times the recommended dose of heparin, a drug used to prevent IV catheters from clotting. The dosage was high enough to cause severe bleeding and death if left untreated. [155]

Infant care, famous parents, renowned hospital. "How could such a thing happen?" you may ask. That is what the Patient Safety and Quality Improvement Act of 2005 is in place to discover.

Drug iatrogenesis may also include anesthesia. Fatal anesthesia errors still occur. Major complications of spinals and epidurals include damage to nerves or the spinal cord by infection (meningitis and abscess), bleeding and blood clots (hematoma), direct damage to the nerves (needle injury or chemical injury) and poor blood supply to the spinal cord (ischemia). All can cause permanent nerve injury including paralysis. A further complication occurs when a "drug switch" or "route switch" occurs: either the wrong drug is delivered as an epidural or spinal (drug switch) or a drug that should have been administered intravenously is used in as an epidural or spinal, or vice versa (route switch). The sensitivity of the nervous system and the type of drugs used means these mistakes can be fatal.[156]

> Although anesthesia is considered very safe, it is not risk free. . . . Uncommon complications include chest infections and difficulty breathing, damage to teeth, lips or tongue, and awareness under general anesthesia. . . . The rare and very rare complications of anesthesia include damage

to the eyes, serious allergic reactions to medications, nerve damage, equipment failure and death. . . .

Deaths caused solely by anesthesia are very rare, and are usually the result of several serious complications together [such as allergies], your previous medical conditions, your body size, your surgical procedure, and your habits like smoking, [all of which may] influence the risks of certain complications. . . . Risk cannot be completely avoided, but the combination of your anesthesia professional's training, modern [sterilized] equipment used to deliver anesthesia and monitor your condition, and modern medications have made anesthesia a much safer procedure in recent years.[157]

Medication Errors

A survey of a 1992 national pharmacy database found a total of 429,827 medication errors in 1,081 hospitals. Medication errors occurred in 5.22% of patients admitted to these hospitals each year. The authors concluded that at least 90,895 patients annually were harmed by medication errors in the US as a whole.[158]

A 2002 study shows that 20% of hospital medications for patients had dosage errors. Nearly 40% of these errors were considered potentially harmful to the patient. In a typical 300-bed hospital, the number of errors per day was 40.[159]

Problems involving patients' medications were even higher the following year. The error rate intercepted by pharmacists in this study was 24%, making the potential minimum number of patients harmed by prescription drugs 417,908.[160]

Adverse Drug Reactions

The Lazarou study[161] analyzed records for prescribed medications for 33 million US hospital admissions in 1994. It discovered 2.2 million serious injuries due to prescribed drugs; 2.1% of inpatients experienced a serious adverse drug reaction, 4.7% of all hospital admissions were due to a serious adverse drug reaction, and fatal adverse drug reactions occurred in 0.19% of inpatients and 0.13% of admissions. The authors estimated that 106,000 deaths occur annually due to adverse drug reactions.

Using a cost analysis from a 2000 study in which the increase in hospitalization costs per patient suffering an adverse drug reaction was $5,483, costs for the Lazarou study's 2.2 million patients with serious drug reactions amounted to $12 billion.[162, 163]

Serious adverse drug reactions commonly emerge after FDA approval of the drugs involved. The safety of new agents cannot be known with certainty until a drug has been on the market for many years.[164]

More recent studies on adverse drug reactions show that the figures may be increasing. A 2003 study followed 400 patients after discharge from a tertiary care hospital setting (requiring highly specialized skills, technology, or support services). Seventy-six patients (19%) had adverse events. Adverse drug events were the most common, at 66% of all events.

The next most common event was procedure-related injuries, at 17%.[165]

In a *New England Journal of Medicine* study, an alarming one in four patients suffered observable side effects from the more than 3.34 billion prescription drugs filled in 2002.[166] One of the doctors who produced the study was interviewed by Reuters and commented, "With these 10-minute appointments, it's hard for the doctor to get into whether the symptoms are bothering the patients."[167]

William Tierney, who editorialized on the *New England Journal* study, wrote, "Given the increasing number of powerful drugs available to care for the aging population, the problem will only get worse." The drugs with the worst record of side effects were selective serotonin reuptake inhibitors (SSRIs), nonsteroidal anti-inflammatory drugs (NSAIDs), and calcium-channel blockers.

Reuters also reported that prior research has suggested that nearly 5% of hospital admissions (over 1 million per year) are the result of drug side effects. But most of the cases are not documented as such. The study found that one of the reasons for this failure is that in nearly two thirds of the cases, doctors could not diagnose drug side effects or the side effects persisted because the doctor failed to heed the warning signs.

In 2004, the world pharmaceutical market did $550 billion in sales; the US market accounted for 48% of that total, which was $248 billion. The US sold nearly half of the world's total of prescription drugs.[168]

Underreporting of Side Effects

Standard medical pharmacology texts admit that relatively few doctors ever report adverse drug reactions to the FDA.[169] The reasons range from not knowing such a reporting system exists to fear of being sued.[170] Yet the public depends on this tremendously flawed system of voluntary reporting by doctors to know whether a drug or a medical intervention is harmful.

Pharmacology texts also will tell doctors how hard it is to separate drug side effects from disease symptoms. Treatment failure is most often attributed to the disease and not the drug or doctor. Doctors are warned, "Probably nowhere else in professional life are mistakes so easily hidden, even from ourselves."[171]

It may be hard to accept, but it is not difficult to understand why only one in twenty side effects is reported to either hospital administrators or the FDA.[172]

If hospitals admitted to the actual number of errors for which they are responsible, which is about twenty times what is reported, they would come under intense scrutiny.[173]

Jerry Phillips, associate director of the FDA's Office of Post Marketing Drug Risk Assessment, confirms this number. "In the broader area of adverse drug reaction data, the 250,000 reports received annually probably represent only 5% of the actual reactions that occur."[174] Dr. Jay Cohen, who has extensively researched adverse drug reactions, notes that because only 5% of adverse drug reactions are reported, there are in fact 5 million medication reactions each year.[175]

Medicating Our Feelings

P atients seeking a more joyful existence and relief from worry, stress, and anxiety are frequently swayed by the messages endlessly displayed on TV and billboards. Often, instead of gaining relief, they fall victim to the myriad iatrogenic side effects of antidepressant medication.

Moreover, a whole generation of antidepressant users has been created from young people growing up on Ritalin®. Medicating young people and modifying their emotions must have some impact on how they learn to deal with their feelings. They learn to equate coping with drugs rather than with their inner resources. As adults, these medicated youth reach for alcohol, drugs, or even street drugs to cope.

According to *JAMA*, "Ritalin® acts much like cocaine."[176] Today's marketing of mood-modifying drugs such as Prozac® and Zoloft® makes them not only socially acceptable, but almost a necessity in today's stressful world.

You cannot turn on TV without hearing a pitch for drugs for social anxiety, depression, or lethargy. Note that when they tell you the side effects, they often show a pastoral scene of beauty, or a joyful activity, at the same time, so you will equate the obligatory warning of danger with a pleasant memory.

Doctors (not just consumers) are bombarded with psychoactive pharmaceutical propaganda, so they will prescribe certain drug products:

> In 2006 money from the pharmaceutical industry accounted for about 30 percent of the [American Psychiatric] Association's $62.5 million in financing. About half of that money went to drug advertisements in psychiatric journals and exhibits at the annual meeting, and the other half to sponsor fellowships, conferences and industry symposiums at the annual meeting.[177]

Television Diagnosis

To reach the widest audience possible, drug companies no longer simply target medical doctors with their marketing of antidepressants.

By 1995, drug companies had tripled the amount of money allotted to direct advertising of prescription drugs to consumers. The majority of this money is spent on seductive television ads. From 1996 to 2000, spending rose from $791 million to nearly $2.5 billion.[178] This $2.5 billion represents only 15% of the total pharmaceutical advertising budget.

While the drug companies maintain that direct-to-consumer advertising is educational, Dr. Sidney M. Wolfe of the Public Citizen Health Research Group in Washington, DC, argues that the public often is misinformed about these ads.[179] People want what they see on television and are told to go to their doctors for a prescription. Doctors in private practice either acquiesce to their patients' demands for these drugs or spend valuable time trying to talk patients out of unnecessary drugs.

Dr. Wolfe remarks that one important study found that people mistakenly believe that the "FDA reviews all ads before they are released and allows only the safest and most effective drugs to be promoted directly to the public."[180]

In 2004, pharmaceutical manufacturers spent an estimated $4.15 billion on direct-to-consumer advertising, according to IMS Health.[181] There are those who surmise that consumers are paying for these expensive ads when they buy medications that cost much more than they are worth.

A finding of a national survey of 643 physicians by Harvard's Dr. Joel Weissman, et al., found that "direct-to-consumer advertising (DTCA) led patients to seek unnecessary treatments."[182]

In 2004, Americans spent $188.5 billion on prescription medications, which was more than 4½ times the $40.3 billion spent in 1990.[183]

Dr. David Graham of the FDA's Center for Drug Evaluation and Research warns:

> Direct-to-consumer advertising in general is a great disservice to the American people. We see wonderful ads of people demonstrating their health, whether they're skating across the ice or doing their Tai Chi. Madison Avenue knows that a picture is worth

a thousand words, so they convey an image, a message, and it makes an impression on patients and on physicians. It creates needs or desires where there really isn't a need or a desire.

There was a recent study in the *Journal of The American Medical Association* that showed that if patients mentioned a drug that they've seen on television to their physician they were much more likely to be prescribed that drug by the doctor. Drug companies know this. That's why they do it. . . . Clearly, direct-to-consumer advertising does not serve the American people well.[184]

How Do We Know Drugs Are Safe?

Another aspect of scientific medicine that the public takes for granted is the testing of new drugs. Drugs generally are tested on individuals who are fairly healthy and not on other medications that could interfere with findings. But when these new drugs are declared "safe" and enter the drug prescription books, they are naturally going to be used by people who are on a variety of other medications and have a lot of other health problems. Then a new phase of drug testing called "post-approval" comes into play, which is the documentation of side effects once drugs hit the market.

In one very telling report, the federal government's General Accountability Office "found that of the 198 drugs approved by the FDA between 1976 and 1985 . . . 102 (or 51.5%) had serious post-approval risks. . . . The serious post-approval risks [included] heart failure, myocardial infarction, anaphylaxis, respiratory depression and arrest, seizures, kidney and liver failure, severe blood disorders, birth defects and fetal toxicity, and blindness."[185]

NBC News's investigative show *Dateline* wondered if your doctor is moonlighting as a drug company representative. After a year-long investigation, NBC reported that because doctors can legally prescribe any drug to any patient for any condition, drug companies heavily promote "off-label"—that is, frequently inappropriate and untested uses of these medications—

even though these drugs are approved only for the specific indications for which they have been tested.[186]

The leading causes of adverse drug reactions are antibiotics (17%), cardiovascular drugs (17%), chemotherapy (15%), and analgesics and anti-inflammatory agents (15%).[187]

Drugs Pollute Our Water Supply

We have reached the point of saturation with prescription drugs. Every body of water tested contains measurable drug residues. The tons of antibiotics used in animal farming, which run off into the water table and surrounding bodies of water, are conferring antibiotic resistance to germs in sewage, and these germs also are found in our water supply. Flushed down our toilets are tons of drugs and drug metabolites that also find their way into our water supply. We have no way to know the long-term health consequences of ingesting a mixture of drugs and drug-breakdown products. These drugs represent another level

of iatrogenic disease that we are unable to completely measure.[188–196]

Drug Companies Fined

Periodically, the FDA fines a drug manufacturer when its abuses are too glaring and
impossible to cover up. In May 2002, the *Washington Post* reported that Schering–Plough
Corp., the maker of Claritin®, was to pay a $500
million fine to the FDA for quality-control problems at four of its factories.[197] The indictment
came after the Public Citizen Health Research
Group, led by Dr. Sidney Wolfe, called for a crim-
inal investigation of Schering–Plough, charging
that the company distributed albuterol asthma
inhalers even though it knew the units were
missing the active ingredient.

The FDA tabulated infractions involving 125
products, or 90% of the drugs made by Scher-
ing-Plough since 1998. Besides paying the fine,
the company was forced to halt the manufacture
of 73 drugs or suffer another $175 million fine.
Schering–Plough's news releases told another

story, assuring consumers that they should still feel confident in the company's products.

This large settlement served as a warning to the drug industry about maintaining strict manufacturing practices and has given the FDA more clout in dealing with drug company compliance. According to the *Washington Post* article, a federal appeals court ruled in 1999 that the FDA could seize the profits of companies that violate "good manufacturing practices." Since that time, Abbott Laboratories has paid a $100 million fine for failing to meet quality standards in the production of medical test kits, while Wyeth Laboratories paid $30 million in 2000 to settle accusations of poor manufacturing practices.

4

Problems with Specific Classes of Drugs

Antibiotics

CCORDING TO WILLIAM AGGER, MD, DIRECTOR of microbiology and chief of infectious disease at Gundersen Lutheran Medical Center in La Crosse, WI, 30 million pounds of antibiotics are used in America each year.[198] Of this amount, 25 million pounds are used in animal husbandry and 23 million pounds are used to try to prevent disease and promote growth. Only 2 million pounds are given for specific animal infections. Dr. Agger reminds us that low concentrations of antibiotics are measurable in many of our foods and in various waterways around the world, much of it seeping in from animal farms.

Agger contends that overuse of antibiotics results in food-borne infections that are resistant to antibiotics. Salmonella is found in 20% of ground meat, but the constant exposure of cattle to antibiotics has made 84% of salmonella resistant to at least one antisalmonella antibiotic. Diseased animal food accounts for 80% of salmonellosis in humans, or 1.4 million cases per year. The conventional approach to countering this epidemic is to radiate food to try to kill all organisms while continuing to use the antibiotics that created the problem in the first place. Approximately 20% of chickens are contaminated with *Campylobacter jejuni*, an organism that causes 2.4 million cases of illness annually. Fifty-four percent of these organisms are resistant to at least one anti-*Campylobacter* antimicrobial agent.

Denmark banned growth-promoting antibiotics beginning in 1999, which cut their use by more than half within a year, from 453,200 to

195,800 pounds. A report from Scandinavia found that removing antibiotic growth promoters had no or minimal effect on food production costs. Agger warns that the current crowded, unsanitary methods of animal farming in the US support constant stress and infection, and are geared toward high antibiotic use.

In the US, over 3 million pounds of antibiotics are used every year on humans. With a population of 284 million Americans, this amount is enough to give every man, woman, and child 10 teaspoons of pure antibiotics per year. Agger says that exposure to a steady stream of antibiotics has altered pathogens such as *Streptococcus pneumoniae*, *Staphylococcus aureus*, and various *Enterococci*, to name a few.

Almost half of patients with upper respiratory tract infections in the US still receive antibiotics from their doctors,[199] which is inappropriate in most cases. In Germany, the prevalence of systemic antibiotic use in children aged 0–6 years was 42.9%.[200]

Data obtained from nine US health insurers on antibiotic use in 25,000 children from

1996 to 2000 found that rates of antibiotic use decreased. Antibiotic use in children aged three months to under three years decreased 24%, from 2.46 to 1.89 antibiotic prescriptions per patient per year. For children aged three to under six years, there was a 25% reduction, from 1.47 to 1.09 antibiotic prescriptions per patient per year. And for children aged 6 to under 18 years, there was a 16% reduction, from 0.85 to 0.69 antibiotic prescriptions per patient per year.[201] Despite these reductions, the data indicate that on average, every child in America receives 1.22 antibiotic prescriptions annually.

Group A beta-hemolytic streptococci is the only common cause of sore throat that requires antibiotics, with penicillin and erythromycin the only recommended treatment. Ninety percent of sore throat cases, however, are viral. Antibiotics were used in 73% of the estimated 6.7 million adult annual visits for sore throat in the US between 1989 and 1999. Furthermore, patients treated with antibiotics were prescribed non-recommended broad-spectrum antibiotics in 68% of visits. This period saw a significant increase in the use of newer, more expensive broad-spectrum antibiotics and a decrease in use of the recommended antibiotics penicillin and erythromycin.[202] Antibiotics being prescribed in 73% of sore throat cases instead of the recommended 10% resulted in a total of 4.2 million unnecessary antibiotic prescriptions for sore throats alone from 1989 to 1999.

In September 2003, the CDC re-launched a program started in 1995 called "Get Smart: Know When Antibiotics Work."[203] This $1.6 million campaign is designed to educate patients about the overuse and inappropriate use of antibiotics. Most people involved with alternative medicine have known about the dangers of antibiotic overuse for decades. Finally, the government is focusing on the problem, yet it is spending only a miniscule amount of money on an iatrogenic epidemic that is costing billions of dollars and thousands of lives. The CDC warns that 90% of upper respiratory infections, including children's ear infections, are viral and that antibiotics do not treat viral infection. More than 40% of prescriptions for antibiotics written each year in physicians' offices are inappropriate.[204, 205] Using antibiotics when not needed can lead to the development of deadly strains of bacteria that are resistant to drugs.[206]

The CDC, however, seems to be blaming patients for misusing antibiotics even though they are available only by prescription from physicians. According to Dr. Richard Besser, then head of the "Get Smart" program to educate patients about proper antibiotic use, "Programs that have just targeted physicians have not worked. Direct-to-consumer advertising of drugs is to blame in some cases." Besser says the program "teaches patients and the general public that antibiotics are precious resources that must be used correctly if we want to have them around when we need them. Hopefully, as a result of this campaign, patients will feel more comfortable asking their doctors for the best care for their illnesses, rather than asking for antibiotics."[207]

What constitutes the "best care"? The CDC does not elaborate and ignores the latest research on the dozens of nutraceuticals that have been scientifically proven to treat viral infections and boost immune-system function. Will doctors recommend garlic, vitamin C, lactoferrin, elderberry, vitamin A, zinc, or DHEA? Probably not. The CDC's commonsense recommendations that most people follow anyway include getting proper rest, drinking plenty of fluids, and using a humidifier.

The pharmaceutical industry claims it supports limiting the use of antibiotics. The drug company Bayer sponsors a program called "Operation Clean Hands" through an organization called LIBRA.[208] The CDC also is involved in trying to minimize antibiotic resistance, but nowhere in its publications is there any reference to the role of nutraceuticals in boosting the immune system, or to the thousands of journal articles that support this approach. This tunnel vision and refusal to recommend the available non-drug alternatives is unfortunate when the CDC is desperately trying to curb the overuse of antibiotics.

The AHRQ reports that currently, "The most common HAI [healthcare-associated infection] agent is methicillin-resistant *Staphylococcus aureus* (MRSA)."[209]

NSAIDS

It is not only the US that is plagued by iatrogenesis. A survey of more than 1,000 French general practitioners (GPs) tested their basic pharmacological knowledge and practice in prescribing NSAIDs, which rank first among commonly prescribed drugs for serious adverse reactions. The study results suggest that GPs do not have adequate knowledge of these drugs and are unable to effectively manage adverse reactions.[210]

A cross-sectional survey of 125 patients attending specialty pain clinics in South London found that possible iatrogenic factors such as "over-investigation, inappropriate information, and advice given to patients as well as misdiagnosis, over-treatment, and inappropriate prescription of medication were common."[211]

In 2003, J.S. Hochman, MD, Executive Director of the National Foundation for the Treatment of Pain, referring to NSAID-related deaths as a "silent epidemic," wrote:

> It has been estimated conservatively that 16,500 NSAID-related deaths

occur among patients with rheumatoid arthritis or osteoarthritis every
year in the United States. This figure is
similar to the number of deaths from
the acquired immunodeficiency syndrome and considerably greater than
the number of deaths from multiple
myeloma, asthma, cervical cancer, or
Hodgkin's disease.[212]

Over 66,000 people were killed over a 10-year
period during the Vietnam War. More people
are killed by NSAIDs in one year (16,500 deaths)
than were killed in any two years of the Vietnam
War. In ten years, NSAIDS kills 165,000 people.
NSAIDS kills 2.5 times as many people in a ten-
year period as were killed in the ten years of the
Vietnam War.

In 2003, the *British Medical Journal* warned
that women who took NSAIDs—"painkillers like
Advil®, Motrin®, and Naprosyn®—had an 80 percent higher risk of miscarriage than women who
avoided these medications."[213] "The risk increased
if such painkillers were taken shortly before or
after conception, or for longer than one week."[214]

On September 30, 2004, Merck announced "a voluntary worldwide withdrawal of Vioxx® (Rofecoxib), its arthritis and acute pain medication." Merck announces voluntary worldwide withdrawal of Vioxx®[215] "due to safety concerns of an increased risk of cardiovascular events (including heart attack and stroke) in patients on rofecoxib. Rofecoxib is a prescription COX-2 selective, non-steroidal anti-inflammatory drug (NSAID) that was approved by the FDA in May 1999."[216] "It was later approved for the relief of the signs and symptoms of rheumatoid arthritis in adults and children."[217] This means that children were exposed to this dangerous drug.

The Lancet carried the following article in its first issue of December 2004, "Risk of cardiovascular events and rofecoxib: cumulative meta-analysis," which finds that "rofecoxib should have been withdrawn several years earlier. The reasons why manufacturer and drug licensing authorities did not continuously monitor and summarize the accumulating evidence need to be clarified."[218]

The NSAID "Vioxx® was withdrawn after evidence came to light that it almost doubled the risk of heart attacks and stroke in people who had been taking it for 18 months."[219] FDA researcher Dr. David Graham, testifying before the US Senate, estimated 88,000 to 138,000 Americans had heart attacks or strokes as a side effect from Vioxx®. "Of these," Graham said, "30–40% probably died."[220] "That would be an estimated 27,000 to 55,000 preventable deaths attributed to Vioxx®."[221]

Dr. Graham continues his Senate testimony, "If there were an average of 150 to 200 people on an aircraft, this range of 88,000 to 138,000 would be the rough equivalent of 500 to 900 aircraft dropping from the sky. This translates to 2–4 aircraft every week, week in and week out, for the past 5 years."[222]

Cancer Chemotherapy

In 1989, German biostatistician Ulrich Abel, PhD, wrote a monograph entitled "Chemotherapy of Advanced Epithelial Cancer." It was later published in shorter form in a peer-reviewed medical journal.[223] Abel presented a comprehensive analysis of clinical trials and publications representing over 3,000 articles examining the value of cytotoxic chemotherapy on advanced epithelial cancer.

Epithelial cancer is the type of cancer with which we are most familiar, arising from epithelium found in the lining of body organs such as the breast, prostate, lung, stomach, and bowel. From these sites, cancer usually infiltrates adjacent tissue and spreads to the bone, liver, lung, or brain. With his exhaustive review, Abel concluded there is no direct evidence that chemotherapy prolongs survival in most patients with advanced carcinoma.

According to Abel, "Many oncologists take it for granted that response to therapy prolongs survival, an opinion which is based on a fallacy and which is not supported by clinical studies." Over a decade after Abel's exhaustive review of chemotherapy, there seems no decrease in its use for advanced carcinoma. For example, when conventional chemotherapy and radiation have not worked to prevent metastases in breast cancer, high-dose chemotherapy (HDC) along with stem-cell transplant (SCT) is the treatment of choice. In March 2000, however, results from the largest multi-center randomized controlled trial conducted thus far showed that, compared to a prolonged course of monthly conventional-dose chemotherapy, HDC and SCT were of no benefit,[224] with even a slightly lower survival rate for the HDC/SCT group.

Serious adverse effects occurred more often in the HDC group than in the standard-dose group. One treatment-related death (within 100 days of therapy) was recorded in the HDC group, but none was recorded in the conventional chemotherapy group. The women in this trial were highly selected as having the best chance to respond.

Unfortunately, no all-encompassing follow-up study such as Dr. Abel's exists to indicate whether there has been any improvement in cancer-survival statistics since 1989. In fact, research should be conducted to determine whether chemotherapy itself is responsible for secondary cancers instead of progression of the original disease. We continue to question why well-researched alternative cancer treatments are not used.

Until now, the extent to which chemotherapy tortures young patients, formerly thought to be strong enough to withstand the toxicity, was unknown.

On August 16, 2006, Harvard Medical School-affiliated Drs. Michael J. Hassett, A. James O'Malley, Juliana R. Pakes, Joseph P. Newhouse, and Craig C. Earle published, "Frequency and Cost of Chemotherapy-Related Serious Adverse Effects in a Population Sample of Women With Breast Cancer" in the *Journal of the National Cancer Institute*.[225] The authors acknowledge that "breast cancer is the most common indication for chemotherapy among women in the United States, and chemotherapy drugs are the leading cause of serious drug-related adverse effects among women with breast cancer," but the authors suggest that studies in older women cannot be extrapolated to the general population. This, therefore, is the first study of chemotherapy-related serious adverse effects in a population-based sample of younger women with breast cancer. 12,239 women 63 years of age or younger with newly diagnosed breast cancer participated in the study. ("A drug-related serious adverse effect has been defined as any untoward medical occurrence that is related to drug use and results in death or significant disability/incapacity, requires hospital admission or prolongation of existing hospital stay, or is life threatening.") Several of the adverse effects are:

- dehydration or electrolyte disorders (potentially fatal);
- fatigue;
- dizziness;
- nausea;
- diarrhea;
- emesis;
- bronchitis (potentially fatal);
- pneumonia (potentially fatal);
- flu (potentially fatal);
- kidney infection (potentially fatal);
- other infections (potentially fatal);
- shock (potentially fatal);
- fever;

- malnutrition;
- anemia (potentially fatal);
- deep-vein thrombosis or pulmonary embolism (potentially fatal);
- fractures and dislocations;
- emphysema (potentially fatal);
- asthma (potentially fatal);
- renal failure (potentially fatal);
- thyroid disorders, including goiter (potentially fatal); and
- headaches, including migraines.

Prior to this study, it was believed that women over age 65 could be expected to have comorbid conditions that would make them more susceptible to adverse side effects of chemotherapy, but that the younger population could survive the toxicity. The authors conclude that "breast cancer chemotherapy may cause more patient suffering and higher healthcare costs than previously estimated."[226]

They emphasize that clinical trials of new drugs are often inadequate to accurately show experiences of the general population. They warn:

Although clinical trials of new drug therapies provide some information regarding the number and nature of serious adverse effects, reports of these complications are frequently inadequate and may not accurately reflect the experiences of the general population. Indeed, recent and widely publicized cases have demonstrated that serious adverse effects that are not fully appreciated during early clinical trials can appear after a drug is approved by the US Food and Drug Administration (FDA) and used by the public. In fact, one study of serious adverse effects identified after FDA approval found that 22 cancer drugs had been linked with 25 serious adverse effects between 2000 and 2002.[227]

The authors conclude that their findings "have important implications for quality of life and could affect decisions regarding [risks of] therapy."

A 2004 pioneer overview study, "The Contribution of Cytotoxic Chemotherapy to 5-year Survival in Adult Malignancies," by Drs. Graeme

Morgan, Robyn Ward, and Michael Barton in *Clinical Oncology* reports that "The overall contribution of curative and adjuvant cytotoxic chemotherapy to 5-year survival in adults was estimated to be . . . 2.1% in the USA."[228] That is, only 2.1% of patients treated with cytotoxic chemotherapy for various malignancies survive for 5 years as a result of chemotherapy. They note that their estimate of benefit is statistically generous, using the "upper limit of effectiveness," and "the benefit of cytotoxic chemotherapy may have been overestimated for cancers of esophagus, stomach, rectum, and brain." The authors refer to "the minimal impact of cytotoxic chemotherapy on 5-year survival, and the lack of any major progress over the last 20 years."

5

An Honest Look at the Failures of American Healthcare

Unnecessary Surgical Procedures

N 1974, 2.4 MILLION UNNECESSARY SURGERIES WERE performed, resulting in 11,900 deaths at a cost of $3.9 billion.[229, 230] In 2001, 7.5 million unnecessary surgical procedures were performed, resulting in 37,136 deaths at a cost of $122 billion (using 1974 dollars).[231, 232]

It is very difficult to obtain accurate statistics when studying unnecessary surgery. In 1989, Leape wrote that perhaps 30% of controversial surgeries—which include cesarean section, tonsillectomy, appendectomy, hysterectomy, gastrectomy for obesity, breast implants, and elective breast implants[233]—are unnecessary.

In 1974, the Congressional Committee on Interstate and Foreign Commerce held hearings on unnecessary surgery. It found that 17.6% of recommendations for surgery were not confirmed by a second opinion. The House Subcommittee on Oversight and Investigations extrapolated these figures and estimated that, on a nationwide basis, there were 2.4 million unnecessary surgeries performed annually, resulting in 11,900 deaths at an annual cost of $3.9 billion.[234]

According to the Healthcare Cost and Utilization Project in the Agency for Healthcare Research and Quality,[235] in 2001 the 50 most common medical and surgical procedures were performed approximately 41.8 million times in the US. Using the 1974 House Subcommittee on Oversight and Investigations' figure of 17.6% as the percentage of unnecessary surgical procedures, and extrapolating from the death rate in 1974, there were nearly 7.5 million (7,489,718) unnecessary procedures and a death rate of 37,136, at a cost of $122 billion (using 1974 dollars). In 1995, researchers conducted a similar analysis of back surgery procedures, using the 1974 "unnecessary surgery percentage" of 17.6%. Testifying before the Department of Veterans Affairs, they estimated that of the 250,000 back surgeries performed annually in the US at a hospital cost of $11,000 per patient, the total number of unnecessary back surgeries approaches 44,000, costing as much as $484 million.[236]

Like prescription drug use driven by television advertising, unnecessary surgeries are escalating. Media-driven surgery such as gastric bypass for obesity "modeled" by Hollywood celebrities seduces obese people into thinking this route is safe and sexy.

Unnecessary surgeries have even been marketed on the Internet.[237] A study in Spain declares that 20–25% of total surgical practice represents unnecessary operations.[238] According to data from the National Center for Health Statistics for 1979 to 1984, the total number of surgical procedures increased 9% while the number of surgeons grew 20%. The study notes that the large increase in the number of surgeons was not accompanied by a parallel increase in the number of surgeries performed, and expressed concern about an excess of surgeons to handle the surgical caseload.[239]

From 1983 to 1994, however, the incidence of the ten most commonly performed surgical procedures jumped 38%, to 7,929,000 from 5,731,000 cases. By 1994, cataract surgery was the most common procedure, with more than two million operations, followed by cesarean section (858,000 procedures) and inguinal hernia operations (689,000 procedures). Knee arthroscopy procedures increased 153% while prostate surgery declined 29%.[240]

The list of iatrogenic complications from surgery is as long as the list of procedures themselves. One study examined catheters that were inserted to deliver anesthetic into the epidural space around the spinal nerves for lower cesarean section, abdominal surgery, or prostate surgery. In some cases, nonsterile technique during catheter insertion resulted in serious infections, even leading to limb paralysis.[241]

In one review of the literature, the authors found "a significant rate of overutilization of coronary angiography, coronary artery surgery, cardiac pacemaker insertion, upper gastrointestinal endoscopies, carotid endarterectomies, back surgery, and pain-relieving procedures."[242]

A 1987 *JAMA* study found the following significant levels of inappropriate surgery: 17% of coronary angiography procedures, 32% of carotid endarterectomy procedures, and 17% of upper gastrointestinal tract endoscopy procedures.[243]

Based on the Healthcare Cost and Utilization Project (HCUP) statistics provided by the government for 2001, 697,675 upper gastrointestinal endoscopies (usually entailing biopsy) were performed, as were 142,401 endarterectomies and 719,949 coronary angiographies.[244]

Extrapolating the *JAMA* study's inappropriate surgery rates to 2001 produces 118,604 unnecessary endoscopy procedures, 45,568 unnecessary endarterectomies, and 122,391 unnecessary coronary angiographies. These are all forms of medical iatrogenesis.

While some 12,000 deaths occur each year from unnecessary surgeries, results from the few studies that have measured unnecessary surgery directly indicate that for some highly controversial operations, the proportion of unwarranted surgeries could be as high as 30%.[245]

High Mortality Rates

It is instructive to know the mortality rates associated with various medical and surgical procedures. Although we must sign release forms when we undergo any procedure, many of us are in denial about the true risks involved; because medical and surgical procedures are so commonplace, they often are seen as both necessary and safe. Unfortunately, allopathic medicine itself is a leading cause of death, as well as the most expensive way to die.

Perhaps the words "healthcare" confer the illusion that medicine is about health. Allopathic medicine is not a purveyor of healthcare but of disease care. The HCUP figures are instructive,[246] but the computer program that calculates annual mortality statistics for all US hospital discharges is only as good as the codes entered into the system. In email correspondence, HCUP indicated that the mortality rates for each procedure indicated only that someone undergoing that procedure died either from the procedure or from some other cause.

Thus, there is no way of knowing exactly how many people die from a particular procedure. While codes for "poisoning and toxic effects of drugs" and "complications of treatment" do exist, the mortality figures registered in these categories are very low and do not correlate with what is known from research such as the 1998 *JAMA* study[247] that estimated an average of 106,000 prescription medication deaths per year. No codes exist for adverse drug side effects, surgical mishaps, or other types of medical error. Until such codes exist, the true mortality rates tied to medical error will remain buried in the general statistics.

A study supported by the Agency for Healthcare Research and Quality that analyzed data from nearly 3 million operations between 1985 and 2004 found that 1 in 112,994 surgeries occurred at the wrong surgical site. Other studies have reported incidence rates up to five times higher, and because not all sentinel events are reported, these figures are likely underestimated. . . .

Wrong-site surgery results in devastating consequences for the patient in terms of morbidity and mortality, as well as negative financial consequences for surgeons and hospitals. For example, studies have shown that 79 percent of wrong-site eye surgeries and 84 percent of wrong-site orthopedic surgeries result in malpractice claims.[248]

Since 2004, surgeons have been required by the Joint Commission [Universal Protocol for

Preventing Wrong Site, Wrong Procedure, Wrong Person Surgery]* to mark the surgical site while consulting with the patient before surgery. Nevertheless, wrong-site surgeries persist at low but unacceptable rates, leading to devastating consequences for those affected. Wrong-site surgeries occur due to a lack of formal systems that ensure compliance with surgical site marking requirements.[249]

Wrong Site, Wrong Procedure, Wrong Person Surgery is not the only iatrogenic surgery that can induce death. The Office of the Chief Medical Examiner of New York City had a mortuary museum started, in part, for the purpose of medical education and iatrogenic reform by innovative NYC Chief Medical Examiner Milton Helpern, MD (CME 1954–1973), based on autopsies performed there. (This museum was later transferred to the Armed Forces Institute of Pathology in Washington, DC).

---

* The Joint Commission's Universal Protocol for Preventing Wrong Site, Wrong Procedure, Wrong Person Surgery [updated version, effective January 1, 2009] is available at http://www.jointcommission.org/PatientSafety/UniversalProtocol/; accessed February 1, 2009.

There is a particularly chilling exhibit in this collection. It is simply a surgical clamp and a large surgical gauze pad, with a descriptive case card. This is a true medical history. A thirty-five-year-old woman entered a hospital in New York for an appendectomy. Postoperative recovery was uneventful, and she was discharged to go home on the eighth day after her operation. The next morning she phoned her surgeon to complain about abdominal cramps. He prescribed routine mild medication, reassuring her that there was nothing to worry about. When the pain persisted, she consulted a second doctor, who diagnosed an "acute intestinal obstruction," and admitted her to another hospital as an emergency case. The second hospital was far away from the first, and a different surgeon performing the second operation discovered that the first surgeon had failed to remove a surgical clamp from the patient's abdomen. Some coils of the small intestine had become entwined with the clamp, resulting in gangrene. The second surgeon removed the gangrenous section of intestine, sewed together the two healthy ends, and closed that incision.[250]

The patient's postoperative course after the second surgery was marked by failure of the incision wound to heal, with accompanying fever. A diagnosis of peritonitis was made. The "wonder" drugs were not yet in use; in two days the patient was dead. The cause of death registered by the medical examiner's office was "septic peritonitis due to the presence of a foreign body." The autopsy had revealed that the second surgeon in the second hospital had left a large surgical gauze pad in the abdominal cavity during the operation that he was performing to remove the metal clamp that had been left by the first negligent surgeon. Surgical malpractice has been documented for many years, but it has not been eliminated.

If you think that might just be a surgical horror story that cannot occur today, then you may be unfamiliar with current medical malpractice case law. The January 2009 article on InjuryBoard.com, "Virginia Has Special Medical Malpractice Law on Retained Surgical Towels," states, "Obviously the hospital and doctor are not supposed to leave things in you, but it is not uncommon for these retained surgical device cases to arise."[251]

Often the patient will go months if not longer before coming to realize that they have some medical equipment like a surgical towel or lap sponge still inside their abdomen after an operation. What typically happens is that the object becomes infected or blocks up some bodily function causing pain. Eventually the patient will get an X-ray or other diagnostic test which will show that something foreign is inside their body cavity. Realizing that there was not a proper accounting of medical supplies done in the operating room may take some time.

The surgeon will typically blame the hospital staff for their failure to do the towel and sponge count and they will in turn point the finger back at him for being the captain of the ship who let something bad happen on his watch and under his command. Both healthcare providers will try to say that maybe the patient herself did something wrong or isn't as hurt as she claims despite what is typically a very bad period of pain and the need for at least one more operation to go in and remove the surgical towel or sponge from the patient's body.[252]

And the *Philadelphia Enquirer* recently reported:

A medical team left behind an unwanted memento in Donald Gable's chest . . . : a two-foot-long guide wire. "I was flabbergasted," said Gable, who developed a blood clot and had to be hospitalized again after the wire was removed. "That thing could have penetrated my vein, and I could have bled to death."

Doctors reviewed the X-rays at least six times before his discharge and did not spot the wire, according to Gable's suit. A doctor discovered the wire when Gable returned for a routine follow-up.

About 80 times a year in the Philadelphia region [alone], the tools of surgery—gauze, scalpels, needles, retractors and the like—are found left behind in patients.

A woman set off an airport metal detector in 2002 because of a . . . ruler-length instrument left inside her abdomen. "There is absolutely no reason for these to occur," said Philadelphia lawyer Paul Lauricella, who won a $2.5 million verdict in a foreign-body case against Frankford Hospital. . . . A 15-inch-square towel had been left in his client's abdomen for three weeks. "All you have to do [to prevent them] is be able to count."

Gauze pads that sop up blood—the most common items left behind—have been tagged with a special strip since the mid-1950s, making them stand out on X-rays. Several area surgeons said they call for such X-rays when counts do not add up.

But the system is far from fool-proof. Chunliu Zhan, a physician and researcher for the federal Agency for Healthcare Research and Quality, found that this mistake occurs 2,700 times a year in the United States. . . . While medical experts have been trying to do away with this error for decades, regulators have been slow to collect cases and study them.

Gauze pads—"sponges" in medical lingo—were left behind twice as often as surgical instruments. Gauze can trap fluid and lead to [potentially fatal] infections, while instruments can puncture an organ. Nearly all require a second operation to be removed [unless the patient expires before the problem is discovered].[253]

The difficulty in tracing deaths resulting from failure to remove sponges and instruments from body cavities is that if a patient who has had surgery due to illness dies, particularly at home, an autopsy is often not required because the death is attributed to the disease, not to an unsuspected foreign object.

These are the kinds of errors that are apparently not being reported by hospitals, laments Josh Goldstein of *The Philadelphia Inquirer*: "'Anybody that is supposed to report close calls and has zero reports is clueless,' said James Bagian, head of the Department of Veterans Affairs' National Center for Patient Safety. 'Management is asleep at the switch and just waiting until they kill someone.'"[254]

There is a two-pronged Surgical Safety Checklist: pre-surgical, as well as post-operative checklist procedures now help to prevent surgical misadventure/death. While it is not an absolute guarantee of safety, it appears to help.

Alex B. Haynes, MD, MPH, of the Harvard School of Public Health and Massachusetts General Hospital, and his colleagues state in their article, "A Surgical Safety Checklist to Reduce Morbidity and Mortality in a Global Population," published in the January 29, 2009, issue of the *New England Journal of Medicine*:

Surgical complications are common and often preventable. We hypothesized that a program to implement a 19-item surgical safety checklist designed to improve team communication and consistency of care would reduce complications and deaths associated with surgery.

Surgical care and its attendant complications represent a substantial burden of disease worthy of attention from the public health community worldwide. Data suggest that at least half of all surgical complications are avoidable.

In 2008, the World Health Organization (WHO) published guidelines identifying multiple recommended practices to ensure the safety of surgical patients worldwide. On the basis of these guidelines, we designed a 19-item checklist intended to be globally applicable and to reduce the rate of major surgical complications.[255]

The New York Times reports in their January 14, 2009, article, "Checklist Reduces Deaths in Surgery" by Eric Nagourney, that "a year after surgical teams at eight hospitals adopted a 19-item checklist, the average patient death rate fell more than 40 percent and the rate of complications fell by about a third."[256]

> [The checklist includes] a requirement that the nursing staff confirm that everything has been sterilized and that all equipment needed is present. Team members must also confirm that the patient has been given antibiotics ahead of the surgery, if called for, to reduce the chance of infection. The checklist also requires team members to verify that there is enough blood on hand if there is a risk of blood loss, that a piece of equipment that measures blood oxygenation is working and that all the medical images needed are present.
>
> Before the operation begins, the checklist calls for the team to confirm

the identity of the patient and the nature of the procedure. Afterward, the doctors and nurses are supposed to review what has been done, including discussing any special steps that need to be taken to aid recovery and confirming no equipment has been left in the patient. . . .

The researchers reviewed the outcome of 7,688 patients who were undergoing noncardiac surgery at the hospitals. About half the patients had surgery before the checklists were adopted, and half after. At the end of the study, the average death rate dropped to 0.8 percent from 1.5 percent, and the average complication rate fell to 7 percent from 11 percent.[257]

Few Medical Procedures Subject to Clinical Trial

In 1978, the US Office of Technology Assessment (OTA) reported, "Only 10–20% of all procedures currently used in medical practice have been shown to be efficacious by controlled trial."[258] In 1995, the OTA compared medical technology in eight countries (Australia, Canada, France, Germany, the Netherlands, Sweden, the UK, and the US) and again noted that few medical procedures in the US have been subjected to clinical trial. It also reported that US infant mortality was high and life expectancy low compared to other developed countries.[259] Legally, the OTA could not be censored, but it could be shut down.

> The congressional Office of Technology Assessment (OTA) closed its doors September 29, 1995. For 23 years, the nonpartisan analytical agency assisted Congress with the complex and highly technical issues that increasingly affect our society.

[Under President Bill Clinton,] the 104th Congress voted to withdraw funding for OTA and its full-time staff of 143 persons, and cover only a skeleton staff and the amount needed for the agency's final closeout.[260]

A January 30, 2009, headline reads, "Hospitals are Still Neglecting to Report Serious Mistakes":

Despite laws in New Jersey and Pennsylvania requiring hospitals to report major medical errors, unanticipated complications, and near misses to state agencies for the purpose of reducing medical mistakes, experts say that hospitals in both states are neglecting to report these kinds of incidents. . . .

In 2007, major medical errors in Pennsylvania included accidentally leaving surgical equipment inside two separate patients at Fox Chase Cancer Center. At Abington Memorial Hospital in 2005, a woman recovering from hip surgery developed open bed sores after being left lying on a bedpan for several hours. In a total violation of state law, none of these incidents was reported by the hospitals responsible.

These individual reporting failures are indicative of a larger trend across Pennsylvania and New Jersey. In 2007, five out of the 80 hospitals in New Jersey neglected to report a single preventable medical error to state agencies. Similarly, a handful of Pennsylvania hospitals reported no serious events and no near misses that could have hurt patients.[261]

The northeast is not the only place in the nation failing to comply:

To put this in perspective, James Conway, a quality expert at the Institute for Healthcare Improvement in Cambridge, Mass., says that on average, 100 patient medical charts document about 40 instances of patient harm. When we compare these statistics to the ones coming in from hospitals, it becomes apparent that underreporting is both pervasive and profound.[262]

There is a "current climate of sloppy enforcement." It is imperative "to make certain that hospitals and doctors are held responsible for serious patient harm,"[263] or more complications and deaths will occur.

Surgical Errors Cost $9 Billion

An October 2003 *JAMA* study from the US government's Agency for Healthcare Research and Quality (AHRQ) documented 32,000 mostly surgery-related deaths costing $9 billion and accounting for 2.4 million extra hospital days in 2000.[264] Data from 20% of the nation's hospitals were analyzed for 18 different surgical complications, including postoperative infections, foreign objects left in wounds, surgical wounds reopening, and postoperative bleeding.

In a press release accompanying the study, AHRQ director Carolyn M. Clancy, MD, noted,

"This study gives us the first direct evidence that medical injuries pose a real threat to the American public and increase the costs of healthcare."[265] According to the study's authors, "The findings greatly underestimate the problem, since many other complications happen that are not listed in hospital administrative data." They added, "The message here is that medical injuries can have a devastating impact on the healthcare system. We need more research to identify why these injuries occur and find ways to prevent them from happening."

The study authors said that improved medical practices, including an emphasis on better hand washing, might help reduce morbidity and mortality rates. In an accompanying *JAMA* editorial, health-risk researcher Dr. Saul Weingart of Harvard's Beth Israel Deaconess Medical Center wrote, "Given their staggering magnitude, these estimates are clearly sobering."[266]

There are two initiatives under way now to address surgical errors directly. They are pre-operative and post-operative.

Unnecessary X-rays

When X-rays were discovered, no one knew the long-term effects of ionizing radiation. In the 1950s, monthly fluoroscopic exams at the doctor's office were routine, and you could even walk into most shoe stores and see X-rays of your foot bones. We still do not know the ultimate outcome of our initial fascination with X-rays.

In those days, it was common practice to X-ray pregnant women to measure their pelvises and make a diagnosis of twins. Finally, a study of 700,000 children born between 1947 and 1964 in 37 major maternity hospitals compared the children of mothers who had received pelvic X-rays during pregnancy to those of mothers who did not. It found that cancer mortality was 40% higher among children whose mothers had been X-rayed.[267]

In present-day medicine, coronary angiography is an invasive surgical procedure that involves snaking a tube through a blood vessel in the groin up to the heart. To obtain useful information,

X-rays are taken almost continuously, with minimum dosages ranging from 460 to 1,580 mrem. The minimum radiation from a routine chest X-ray is 2 mrem. X-ray radiation accumulates in the body, and ionizing radiation used in X-ray procedures has been shown to cause gene mutation. The health impact of this high level of radiation is unknown, and often obscured in statistical jargon such as, "The risk for lifetime fatal cancer due to radiation exposure is estimated to be 4 in 1 million per 1,000 mrem."[268]

Dr. John Gofman has studied the effects of radiation on human health for 45 years. A medical doctor with a PhD in nuclear and physical chemistry, Dr. Gofman worked on the Manhattan Project, discovered uranium–233, and was the first person to isolate plutonium.

In five scientifically documented books, Dr. Gofman provides strong evidence that medical technology—specifically X-rays, CT scans, and mammography and fluoroscopy devices—are a contributing factor to 75% of new cancers. In a nearly 700-page report updated in 2000, "Radiation from Medical Procedures in the Pathogenesis of Cancer and Ischemic Heart Disease: Dose-Response Studies with Physicians per 100,000 Population,"[269] Gofman shows that as the number of physicians increases in a geographical area along with an increase in the number of X-ray diagnostic tests performed, the rate of cancer and ischemic heart disease also increases.

Gofman elaborates that it is not X-rays alone that cause the damage but a combination of health risk factors that include poor diet, smoking, abortions, and the use of birth control pills. Dr. Gofman predicts that ionizing radiation will be responsible for 100 million premature deaths over the next decade.

In his book *Preventing Breast Cancer*, Dr. Gofman notes that breast cancer is the leading cause of death among American women between the ages of 44 and 55. Because breast tissue is highly sensitive to radiation, mammograms can cause cancer.

The danger can be heightened by other factors, including a woman's genetic makeup, pre-existing benign breast disease, artificial menopause, obesity, and hormone imbalance.[270]

The Journal of the National Cancer Institute published the following statements in their 2004 paper, "Full-Body CT Screening: Preventing or Producing Cancer?" by R. Twombly. "Full-body computed tomography (CT) screening may constitute more of a cancer risk than a cancer foil, say researchers who . . . liken the radiation exposure during a single scan to that experienced within miles of a World War II atom bomb explosion."[271]

The September 2004 issue of *Radiology* includes an article by David Brenner, Ph.D., Professor of Radiation Oncology and Public Health at Columbia University in New York.

> [Brenner] estimated the dose of radiation to the lung or stomach from a single full-body CT scan to be 14–21 milligrays (mGy, a unit of absorbed radiation). That corresponds to a dose region—about 1.5 miles from the blast of an atomic bomb—for which there is direct evidence of increased mortality among atomic bomb survivors, Brenner said. The exposure is "equal

to 100 chest X-rays or 100 mammo-grams," he said.[272]

In the last few years, independent companies offering full-body CT scans has doubled. The CT scan is popular with the well-to-do middle-aged and seniors "who are willing to pay an average of $1,000 to ensure that their aging bodies are not harboring tumors or other incipient diseases."[273] They do not know that they may well develop malignant neoplastic disease as a result of the CT scan itself.

Even X-rays for back pain can lead someone into crippling surgery. Dr. John E. Sarno, a well-known New York orthopedic surgeon, found that there is not necessarily any association between back pain and spinal X-ray abnormality. He cites studies of normal people without a trace of back pain whose X-rays indicate spinal abnormalities and of people with back pain whose spines appear to be normal on X-ray.[274] People who happen to have back pain and show an abnormality on X-ray may be treated surgically, sometimes with no change in back pain, worsening of back pain, or even permanent disability.

Moreover, doctors often order X-rays as protection against malpractice claims, to give the impression of leaving no stone unturned. It appears that doctors are putting their own fears before the interests of their patients.

Unnecessary Hospitalization

Nearly 9 million (8,925,033) people were hospitalized unnecessarily in 2001.[275-278] In a study of inappropriate hospitalization, two doctors reviewed 1,132 medical records. They concluded that 23% of all admissions were inappropriate and an additional 17% could have been handled in outpatient clinics. Thirty-four percent of all hospital days were deemed inappropriate and could have been avoided.[279]

The rate of inappropriate hospital admissions in 1990 was 23.5%.[280] In 1999, another study also found an inappropriate admissions rate of 24%, indicating a consistent pattern from 1986 to 1999.[281] The HCUP database indicates that the total number of patient discharges from US hospitals in 2001 was 37,187,641,[282] meaning that almost 9 million people were exposed to unnecessary medical intervention in hospitals and therefore represent almost 9 million potential iatrogenic episodes.[283–286]

Nosocomial Infections

The rate of nosocomial (in-hospital) infections per 1,000 patient days rose from 7.2 in 1975 to 9.8 in 1995, a 36% jump in 20 years. Reports from more than 270 US hospitals showed that the nosocomial infection rate itself had remained stable over the previous 20 years, with approximately 5–6 hospital-acquired infections occurring per 100 admissions. Due to progressively shorter inpatient stays and the increasing number of admissions, however, the number of infections has increased.

It is estimated that in 1995, nosocomial infections cost $4.5 billion and contributed to more than 88,000 deaths, or one death every six minutes.[287] The 2003 incidence of nosocomial mortality is probably higher than in 1995 because of the tremendous increase in antibiotic-resistant organisms. *Morbidity and Mortality Report* found that nosocomial infections cost $5 billion annually in 1999,[288] representing a $0.5 billion increase in just four years. At this rate of increase, the current cost of nosocomial infections would be close to $6 billion, or more.

As mentioned earlier in Table 1 (page 27), the CDC reports that the number of deaths from healthcare-associated infections in hospitals alone has risen to 99,000 per year. Some of these deaths may be due to poor hygiene on the part of physicians.[289, 290]

According to HealthGrades's Second Annual Patient Safety in American Hospitals Report, May 2005:

> If American hospitals were to implement what we know works, many costly complications could be avoided and lives would be saved. For example, we know that washing hands before patient contact is a simple and effective process that is proven to reduce hospital-acquired infection rates.[291]

Outpatient Iatrogenesis

In a 2000 *JAMA* article, Dr. Barbara Starfield presents well-documented facts that are both shocking and unassailable.[292, 293] The US ranks 12th of 13 industrialized countries when judged by 16 health status indicators. Japan, Sweden, and Canada were first, second, and third, respectively. More than 40 million people in the US have no health insurance, and 20–30% of patients receive contraindicated care.

Starfield warned that one cause of medical mistakes is overuse of technology, which may create a "cascade effect" leading to still more treatment. She urges the use of ICD (International Classification of Diseases) codes that have designations such as "Drugs, Medicinal, and Biological Substances Causing Adverse Effects in Therapeutic Use" and "Complications of Surgical and Medical Care" to help doctors quantify and recognize the magnitude of the medical error problem.

Starfield notes that many deaths attributable to medical error today are likely to be coded to indicate some other cause of death. She concludes that against the backdrop of our poor health report card compared to other Western countries, we should recognize that the harmful effects of healthcare interventions account for a substantial proportion of our excess deaths.

Starfield cites Weingart's 2000 article, "Epidemiology of Medical Error," as well as other authors to suggest that between 4% and 18% of consecutive patients in outpatient settings suffer an iatrogenic event leading to:

- 116 million extra physician visits
- 77 million extra prescriptions filled
- 17 million emergency department visits
- 8 million hospitalizations
- 3 million long-term admissions
- 199,000 additional deaths
- $77 billion in extra costs[294]

6

Women's Experience in Medicine

Hysteria

D R. MARTIN CHARCOT (1825–1893) WAS WORLD-renowned, the most celebrated doctor of his time. He practiced in the Paris hospital La Salpetriere. He became an expert in hysteria, diagnosing an average of 10 hysterical women each day, transforming them into "iatrogenic monsters" and turning simple "neurosis" into hysteria.[295] The number of women diagnosed with hysteria and hospitalized rose from 1% in 1841 to 17% in 1883.

"Hysteria" is derived from the Latin *hystera*, meaning uterus. According to Dr. Adriane Fugh-Berman, US medicine has a tradition of excessive medical and surgical interventions on women. Only 100 years ago, male doctors believed that female psychological imbalance originated in the uterus. When surgery to remove the uterus was perfected, it became the "cure" for mental instability, effecting a physical and psychological castration.

Fugh-Berman notes that US doctors eventually disabused themselves of that notion but have continued to treat women very differently than they treat men.[296] She cites the following statistics:

- Thousands of prophylactic mastectomies are performed annually.
- One third of US women have had a hysterectomy before menopause.
- Women are prescribed drugs more frequently than are men.

- Women are given potent drugs for disease prevention, which results in disease substitution due to side effects.

- Fetal monitoring is unsupported by studies and not recommended by the CDC.[297] It confines women to a hospital bed and may result in a higher incidence of cesarean section.[298] (Fetal monitor is also an instrument inadvertently left in body cavity of the mother.)

- Normal processes such as menopause and childbirth have been heavily "medicalized."

- Synthetic hormone replacement therapy (HRT) does not prevent heart disease or dementia, but does increase the risk of breast cancer, heart disease, stroke, and gall bladder attack.[299]

- As many as a third of postmenopausal women use non-natural (synthetic) HRT.[300, 301] This number is important in light of the much-publicized Women's Health Initiative study, which was halted before its completion because of a higher death rate in the synthetic estrogen–progestin (HRT) group.[302]

Hysterectomy

Perhaps the most infamous and often unnecessary surgical procedure is the hysterectomy, especially when performed on women close to menopause, after which many adverse symptoms, such as uterine bleeding, disappear with the natural reduction of estrogen levels.

"Since the 1960s, hysterectomy has been one of the most frequently performed inpatient surgical procedures in the United States, with an estimated 33% of women undergoing a hysterectomy by 60 years of age," according to the CDC.[303] It is clear from these statistics that until the late 1980s (or later), one-third of all women in the US had hysterectomies. It is probable that many more were told to have a hysterectomy (it was "in fashion"), but if they went for a second opinion to a more conservative doctor, skilled at considering their case carefully on an individual basis, they might be told to just go home. It is well known that many of these women lived well into their eighties without the recommended surgery, according to empirical evidence.

The hysterectomy is controversial to this day, but many doctors are more cautious now before they perform these operations that project women into premature menopause, and they will reserve this surgery for life-saving purposes only, not for "comfort" from pain or bleeding. This surgery may place women at greater risk for disease, as it shifts hormonal balance drastically.

Cesarean Section

In 1983, 809,000 cesarean sections (21% of live births) were performed in the US, making it the nation's most common obstetric-gynecologic (ob-gyn) surgical procedure. The second most common ob-gyn operation was hysterectomy (673,000), followed by diagnostic dilation and curettage of the uterus (632,000). In 1983, ob-gyn procedures represented 23% of all surgeries completed in the US.[304]

In 2001, cesarean section was still the most common ob-gyn surgical procedure. Approximately 4 million births occur annually, with 24% (960,000) delivered by cesarean section. In the Netherlands, only 8% of births are delivered by cesarean section. This suggests 640,000 unnecessary cesarean sections—entailing three to four times higher mortality and twenty times greater morbidity than vaginal delivery[305]—are performed annually in the US.

The US cesarean rate rose from just 4.5% in 1965 to 24.1% in 1986. Sakala contends that an "uncontrolled pandemic of medically unnecessary cesarean births is occurring."[306] VanHam reported a cesarean section postpartum hemorrhage rate of 7%, a hematoma formation rate of 3.5%, a urinary tract infection rate of 3%, and a combined postoperative morbidity rate of 35.7% in a high-risk population undergoing cesarean section.[307]

7

Poor Care of the Elderly

Bedsores

OVER 1 MILLION PEOPLE DEVELOP BEDSORES in US hospitals every year. It is a tremendous burden to patients and family, and a $55 billion healthcare burden.[308] Bedsores are preventable with proper nursing care. It is true that 50% of those affected are in a vulnerable age group of over 70.

In the elderly, bedsores carry a fourfold increase in the rate of death.

The mortality rate in hospitals for patients with bedsores is between 23% and 37%.[309] Even if we just take the 50% of people over 70 with bedsores and the lowest mortality at 23%, that gives us a death rate due to bedsores of 115,000. Critics will say that it was the disease or advanced age that killed the patient, not the bedsores, but our argument is that an early death, by denying proper care, deserves to be counted. It is only after counting these unnecessary deaths that we can then turn our attention to fixing the problem.

Malnutrition in Nursing Homes

The General Accountability Office (GAO), a special investigative branch of Congress, cited 20% of the nation's 17,000 nursing homes for violations between July 2000 and January 2002. Many violations involved serious physical injury and death.[310]

A report from the Coalition for Nursing Home Reform states that at least one third of the nation's 1.6 million nursing home residents may suffer from malnutrition and dehydration, which hastens their death. The report calls for adequate nursing staff to help feed patients who are not able to manage a food tray by themselves.[311] It is difficult to place a mortality rate on malnutrition and dehydration.

The coalition report states that compared with well-nourished hospitalized nursing home residents, malnourished residents have a fivefold increase in mortality when they are admitted to a hospital. Multiplying the one third of 1.6 million nursing home residents who are malnourished by a mortality rate of 20%[312, 313] results in 108,800 premature deaths due to malnutrition in nursing homes.

Warehousing Our Elders

One way to measure the moral and ethical fiber of a society is by how it treats its weakest and most vulnerable members. In some cultures, elderly people live out their lives in extended family settings that enable them to continue participating in family and community affairs. American nursing homes, where millions of our elders go to live out their final days, represent the pinnacle of social isolation and medical abuse:

- In America, approximately 1.6 million elderly are confined to nursing homes. By 2050, that number could be 6.6 million.[314, 315]
- Twenty percent of all deaths from all causes occur in nursing homes.[316]
- Hip fractures are the single greatest reason for nursing home admissions.[317]
- Nursing homes represent a reservoir for drug-resistant organisms due to overuse of antibiotics.[318]

Presenting a report he sponsored entitled "Abuse of Residents Is a Major Problem in US Nursing Homes" on July 30, 2001, Rep. Henry Waxman (D–CA) noted that "as a society we will be judged by how we treat the elderly." The report found one third of the nation's approximately 17,000 nursing homes were cited for an abuse violation in a two-year period from

January 1999 to January 2001.[319] According to Waxman, "the people who cared for us deserve better." The report suggests that this known abuse represents only the "tip of the iceberg" and that much more abuse occurs that we are not aware of or ignore.[320] The report found:

- Over 30% of US nursing homes were cited for abuses, totaling more than 9,000 violations.
- Ten percent of nursing homes had violations that caused actual physical harm to residents or worse.
- Over 40% (3,800) of the abuse violations followed the filing of a formal complaint, usually by concerned family members.
- Many verbal abuse violations were found, as were occasions of sexual abuse.
- Incidents of physical abuse causing numerous injuries, such as fractured femurs, hips, elbows, and wrists, also were found.

Dangerously understaffed nursing homes lead to neglect, abuse, overuse of medications, and physical restraints. In 1990, Congress mandated an exhaustive study of nurse-to-patient ratios in nursing homes. The study was finally begun in 1998 and took four years to complete.[321] A spokesperson for the National Citizens' Coalition for Nursing Home Reform commented on the study:

> They compiled two reports of three volumes, each thoroughly documenting the number of hours of care residents must receive from nurses and nursing assistants to avoid painful, even dangerous, conditions such as bedsores and infections. Yet it took the Department of Health and Human Services and Secretary Tommy Thompson only four months to dismiss the report as "insufficient."[322]

Although preventable with proper nursing care, bedsores occur three times more commonly in nursing homes than in acute care or veterans hospitals.[323]

Because many nursing home patients suffer from chronic debilitating conditions, their assumed cause of death often is unquestioned by physicians. Some studies show that as many as 50% of deaths due to restraints, falls, suicide, homicide, and choking in nursing homes may be covered up.[324, 325] It is possible that many nursing home deaths are instead attributed to heart disease. In fact, researchers have found that heart disease may be over-represented in the general population as a cause of death on death certificates by 8–24%. In the elderly, the over-reporting of heart disease as a cause of death is as much as twofold.[326]

When elucidating iatrogenesis in nursing homes, some critics have asked, "To what extent did these elderly people already have life-threatening diseases that led to their premature deaths anyway?" Our response is that if a loved one dies one day, one week, one year, a decade, or two decades prematurely as a result of some medical misadventure, that is still an untimely iatrogenic death. In a legalistic sense perhaps more weight is placed on the loss of many potential years compared to an additional few weeks, but this attitude is not justified in an ethical or moral sense.

That very few statistics exist concerning malnutrition in acute care hospitals and nursing homes demonstrates the lack of concern in this area. While a survey of the literature turns up few US studies, one revealing US study evaluated the nutritional status of 837 patients in a 100-bed subacute care hospital over a 14-month period. The study found only 8% of the patients were well nourished, while 29% were malnourished and 63% were at risk of malnutrition. As a result, 25% of the malnourished patients required readmission to an acute care hospital, compared to 11% of the well nourished patients. The authors concluded that malnutrition reached epidemic proportions in patients admitted to this subacute care facility.[327]

Many studies conclude that physical restraints are an underreported and preventable cause of death. Studies show that compared to no restraints, the use of restraints carries a higher mortality rate and economic burden.[328–330] Studies have found that physical restraints, including bedrails, are the cause of at least 1 in every 1,000 nursing-home deaths.[331–333]

Deaths caused by malnutrition, dehydration, and physical restraints, however, are rarely recorded on death certificates. Several studies reveal that nearly half of the listed causes of death on death certificates for elderly people with chronic or multi-system disease are inaccurate.[334] Although one in five people dies in nursing homes, an autopsy is performed in less than 1% of these deaths.[335]

Overmedicating Seniors

The CDC seems to be focusing on reducing the number of prescriptions to children, but a 2003 study finds over-medication of US elderly. Dr. Robert Epstein, chief medical officer of Medco Health Solutions Inc. (a unit of Merck & Co.), conducted a study in 2003 of drug trends among the elderly.[336] He found that seniors are going to multiple physicians, getting multiple prescriptions, and using multiple pharmacies. Medco oversees drug-benefit plans for more than 60 million Americans, including 6.3 million seniors who received more than 160 million prescriptions.

According to the study, the average senior receives 25 prescriptions each year. Among those 6.3 million seniors, a total of 7.9 million medication alerts were triggered: less than half that number, 3.4 million, were detected in 1999. About 2.2 million of those alerts indicated excessive dosages unsuitable for seniors, and about 2.4 million alerts indicated clinically inappropriate drugs for the elderly.

Reuters interviewed Kasey Thompson, director of the Center on Patient Safety at the American Society of Health System Pharmacists, who noted: "There are serious and systemic problems with poor continuity of care in the United States." He says this study represents "the tip of the iceberg" of a national problem.[337]

According to *Drug Benefit Trends*, the average number of prescriptions dispensed per non-Medicare HMO member per year rose 5.6% from 1999 to 2000, from 7.1 to 7.5 prescriptions. The average number dispensed for Medicare members increased 5.5%, from 18.1 to 19.1 prescriptions.[338] The total number of prescriptions written in the US in 2000 was 2.98 billion, or 10.4 prescriptions for every man, woman, and child.[339]

In a study of 818 residents of residential care facilities for the elderly, 94% were receiving at least one medication at the time of the interview. The average intake of medications was five per resident; the authors noted that many of these drugs were given without a documented diagnosis justifying their use.[340]

Seniors and groups like the American Association of Retired Persons (AARP) have accepted allopathic medicine's overriding assumption that aging and dying in America must be accompanied by drugs in nursing homes and eventual hospitalization.[341] Seniors are given the choice of either high-cost patented drugs or low-cost generic drugs. Drug companies attempt to keep the most expensive drugs on the shelves and suppress access to generic drugs, despite facing stiff fines of hundreds of millions of dollars levied by the federal government.[342, 343] In 2001, some of the world's largest drug companies were fined a record $871 million for conspiring to increase the price of vitamins.[344]

What if some of these chronic diseases are really lifestyle diseases caused by deficiency of essential nutrients, lack of care, inappropriate medication, overmedication, and isolation? This question is extremely important to consider, yet current AARP recommendations for diet and nutrition assume that seniors are getting all the nutrition they need in an average diet. At most, AARP suggests adding extra calcium and a multivitamin and mineral supplement.[345] We would urge AARP to become more involved in prevention of disease, and not to rely so heavily on drugs. We would like to send the same message to the Hemlock Society, which offers euthanasia options to chronically ill people, especially those in severe pain, who may have become depressed. We must look to healing, lifting pain, releasing depression, instead of cashing in granny's chips. Let's also look at the irony of underuse of proper pain medication for patients who really need it.

Ironically, studies do indicate underuse of appropriate pain medication for patients who need it. One study evaluated pain management in a group of 13,625 cancer patients, aged 65 and over, living in nursing homes. While almost 30% of the patients reported pain, more than 25% received no pain-relief medication, 16% received a mild analgesic drug, 32% received a moderate analgesic drug, and 26% received adequate pain-relieving morphine. The authors concluded that older patients and minority patients were more likely to have their pain untreated.[346]

The time has come to set a standard for caring for the vulnerable among us—a standard that goes beyond making sure they are housed and fed, and not openly abused. We must stop looking the other way and we, as a society, must take responsibility for the way in which we deal with those who are unable to care for themselves.

8

Medical Ethics and Conflicts of Interest in Scientific Medicine

JONATHAN QUICK, DIRECTOR OF ESSENTIAL DRUGS and medicines policy for the World Health Organization (WHO), wrote in a WHO bulletin:

> If clinical trials become a commercial venture in which self-interest overrules public interest and desire overrules science, then the social contract which allows research on human subjects in return for medical advances is broken. [347]

As former editor of the *New England Journal of Medicine*, Dr. Marcia Angell struggled to bring greater attention to the problem of commercializing scientific research. In her outgoing editorial entitled "Is Academic Medicine for Sale?" Angell wrote that growing conflicts of interest are tainting science, and called for stronger restrictions on pharmaceutical stock ownership and other financial incentives for researchers: "When the boundaries between industry and academic medicine become as blurred as they are now," Angell wrote, "the business goals of industry influence the mission of medical schools in multiple ways." She did not discount the benefits of research but said a Faustian bargain now existed between medical schools and the pharmaceutical industry.[348]

Angell left the *New England Journal* in June 2000. In June 2002, *The New England Journal of Medicine* announced that it would accept journalists who accept money from drug companies because it was too difficult to find ones who have no ties. Another former editor of the journal, Dr. Jerome Kassirer, said that was not the case and that plenty of researchers are available who do not work for drug companies.[349] According to an ABC News report, pharmaceutical companies spend over $2 billion a year on over 314,000 events attended by doctors.

The ABC News report also noted that a survey of clinical trials revealed that when a drug company funds a study, there is a 90% chance that the drug will be perceived as effective, whereas a non-drug-company-funded study will show favorable results only 50% of the time. It appears that money can't buy you love, but it can buy any "scientific" result desired.

Cynthia Crossen, a staffer for the *Wall Street Journal*, in 1996 published *Tainted Truth: The Manipulation of Fact in America*, a book about the widespread practice of lying with statistics.[350] Commenting on the state of scientific research, she wrote: "The road to hell was paved with the flood of corporate research dollars that eagerly filled gaps left by slashed government research funding." Her data on financial involvement showed that in 1981, the drug industry "gave" $292 million to colleges and universities for research. By 1991, this figure had risen to $2.1 billion.

> Universities have been treading on dangerous ground with their increasingly complex financial ties to industry. . . . They are worried that these things could ultimately affect their tax-free status," Dr. Kassirer said in September 2008.[351]

In September 2008,

> *The Wall Street Journal* reported that Chair of the Senate Finance Committee Sen. Chuck Grassley . . . confronted about 20 universities across the nation, including Brown, Harvard and Stanford for failing to publicize additional grants obtained from drug makers.[352]

The university is not the only venue for pharmaco-gifts. "Right now the public has no way to know whether a doctor's been given money that might affect prescribing habits," Grassley said as he introduced the Physician Payments Sunshine Act for public disclosure of payments to physicians. Sen. Grassley continues:

Payments to a doctor can be big or small. They can be a simple dinner after work or they can add up to tens of thousands and even hundreds of thousands of dollars each year. That's right—hundreds of thousands of dollars for one doctor. It's really pretty shocking. Companies wouldn't be paying this money unless it had a direct effect on the prescriptions doctors write, and the medical devices they use. Patients, of course, are in the dark about whether their doctor is receiving this money.

This practice, and the lack of transparency around it, can obscure the most important question that exists between doctor and patient: what is best for the patient?[353]

"More Studies!"

Scientists claimed there were never enough studies revealing the dangers of DDT and other dangerous pesticides to ban them. They also used this argument for tobacco, claiming that more studies were needed before they could be certain that tobacco really caused lung cancer. Even the American Medical Association (AMA) was complicit in suppressing the results of tobacco research. In 1964, when the Surgeon General's report condemned smoking, the AMA refused to endorse it, claiming a need for more research. What they really wanted was more money, which they received from a consortium of tobacco companies that paid the AMA $18 million over the next nine years, during which the AMA said nothing about the dangers of smoking.[354]

The *Journal of the American Medical Association (JAMA)*, "after careful consideration of the extent to which cigarettes were used by physicians in practice," began accepting tobacco advertisements and money in 1933. State journals such as the *New York State Journal of Medicine* also began to run advertisements for Chesterfield cigarettes that claimed cigarettes are "Just as pure as the water you drink . . . and practically untouched by human hands." In 1948, *JAMA* argued, "More can be said in behalf of smoking as a form of escape from tension than against it . . . there does not seem to be any preponderance of evidence that would indicate the abolition of the use of tobacco as a substance contrary to the public health."[355] Today, scientists continue to use the excuse that more studies are needed before they will support restricting the inordinate use of drugs.

9

Conclusion

What Remains to Be Uncovered

OUR ONGOING RESEARCH WILL CONTINUE TO quantify the morbidity, mortality, and financial loss due to:

- X-ray exposure (mammography, fluoroscopy, CT scans)
- Overuse of antibiotics for all conditions
- Carcinogenic drugs (hormone replacement therapy,* immunosuppressive and prescription drugs)

---

* Part of our ongoing research will be to quantify the mortality and morbidity caused by hormone replacement therapy (HRT) since the 1940s.

- Cancer chemotherapy
- Surgery and unnecessary surgery (cesarean section, radical mastectomy, preventive mastectomy, radical hysterectomy, prostatectomy, cholecystectomies, cosmetic surgery, arthroscopy, etc.)
- Discredited medical procedures and therapies
- Unproven medical therapies
- Outpatient surgery
- Doctors themselves

In December 2000, a government scientific advisory panel recommended that synthetic estrogen be added to the nation's list of cancer-causing agents. HRT, either synthetic estrogen alone or combined with synthetic progesterone, is used by an estimated 13.5 to 16 million women in the US.[356] The aborted Women's Health Initiative Study (WHI) of 2002 showed that women taking synthetic estrogen combined with synthetic progesterone have a higher incidence of blood clots, breast cancer, stroke, and heart disease, with little evidence of osteoporosis reduction or dementia prevention. WHI researchers, who usually never make recommendations except to suggest more studies, advised doctors to be very cautious about prescribing HRT to their patients.[357, 358–362]

Results of the "Million Women Study" on HRT and breast cancer in the UK were published in medical journal *The Lancet* in August 2003. According to lead author Prof. Valerie Beral, director of the Cancer Research UK Epidemiology Unit, "We estimate that over the past decade, use of HRT by UK women aged 50–64 has resulted in an extra 20,000 breast cancers, estrogen-progestagen (combination) therapy accounting for 15,000 of these."[363]

We were unable to find statistics on breast cancer, stroke, uterine cancer, or heart disease caused by HRT used by American women. Because the US population is roughly six times that of the UK, it is possible that 120,000 cases of breast cancer have been caused by HRT in the past decade.

According to the article "Breast Cancer Risk Remains After Stopping HRT," published on March 5, 2008,

Women who took estrogen plus progestin in the Women's Health Initiative (WHI) trial of hormone replacement therapy (HRT) remain at higher risk of breast cancer three years after the trial was stopped, compared with those who took placebo. . . .

Dr. Gerardo Heiss (University of North Carolina, Chapel Hill) and colleagues report their findings in the March 5, 2008 issue of the *Journal of the American Medical Association*. . . . "What was not anticipated was the greater risk of malignancies overall. . . ." said Dr. Heiss.

The WHI trial of estrogen plus progestin included 16,608 postmenopausal women and set out to examine whether conjugated equine estrogens (CEE) plus medroxyprogesterone acetate (MPA) prevented cardiovascular disease and fractures and to examine any associated change in the risk of breast cancer. The trial was stopped prematurely in 2002 when data indicated an increased risk of breast cancer and unexpected, higher risks of stroke, MI, and venous thromboembolism.

In the new analysis, Heiss and colleagues examined the risk/benefit balance of 15,730 of the participants after the trial was stopped in July 2002 out to March 2005. . . . The annualized event rates for the outcome "all cancers" was higher during the postintervention follow-up for the HRT group (1.56% per year) compared with the placebo group (1.26% per year). This was primarily due to a greater risk of invasive breast cancer: 79 women who took HRT developed breast cancer in the postintervention phase compared with 60 who got placebo. . . . "The hormones' effects on breast cancer appear to linger," says Dr. Leslie Ford (National Cancer Institute, Bethesda, MD). . . .

There is some evidence that HRT is associated with decreased survival in women with lung cancer.

Dr Elizabeth G. Nabel (director, National Heart, Lung, and Blood Institute, Bethesda, MD) also warns, "These findings also indicate that women who take estrogen plus progestin continue to be at increased risk of breast cancer, even years after stopping therapy. Today's report confirms the study's primary conclusion that combination hormone therapy should not be used to prevent disease in healthy, postmenopausal women." Heiss agrees: "The balance of the benefits and risks of estrogen plus progestin therapy continues to be unfavorable after stopping therapy," he explained to *HeartWire*. "As such, these findings confirm the results of the WHI study as originally published—this is not a preparation that ought to be used over long periods to prevent chronic disease. That's it in a nutshell.

"Overall, the summary of benefits and risks appears to be unfavorable," Heiss reiterates, "and this suggests that vigilance is required after the use of these preparations. Women should take care of their health and lifestyle. . . ."

The results of the WHI trial [include] increased risks for myocardial infarction, stroke, deep venous thrombosis, and breast cancer associated with active treatment. A global index suggested that the overall risks for hormone therapy outweighed any benefits.[364]

What has yet to be uncovered about this HRT is why the trials continued as long as they did with the women's lives at stake. We do not recommend synthetic hormone replacement therapy.

Summary

The Office of Technology Assessment (OTA) was perhaps the US government's last honest agency that critically reviewed the state of the nation's healthcare system. The purpose of the OTA was to provide Congress with objective and authoritative analysis of complex scientific and technical issues. In its final critical report, the OTA concluded: "There are no mechanisms in place to limit dissemination of technologies, regardless of their clinical value."

Shortly after the OTA released a report that exposed how entrenched financial interests manipulate healthcare practice in the United States, Congress disbanded the OTA.

Someone has said that healthcare is the only business where you keep paying whether you get good results or not. We do not tolerate poor service in the non-medical marketplace, yet we have accepted it for years in healthcare. For years, our nation has avoided responsibility for examining this major health crisis, to our own mounting peril. Now, we have an iatrogenic epidemic. More Americans are dying each year at the hands of medicine than all of our American casualties in the First World War and the Civil War combined.

Why would highly trained medical doctors continue to follow failing protocols year after year, producing negative results? The chemotherapy studies cited in this paper show that the cytotoxicity is damaging the quality of life and often causing death.

The reason the medical establishment can continue to betray the public trust is because there are no sufficient consequences for killing or maiming patients. The physician is rewarded for his *efforts*, not for his results. It is taken for granted that if you have chemotherapy, you will be maimed, and possibly killed. The patient even signs away his or her rights before surgery, so that the surgeon and hospital are protected even if they are negligent.

The proprietary interests connected with these approved protocols make them attractive for physicians and hospitals to follow. The pharmaceutical companies reward physicians who buy and use their drugs. Grants are offered to hospitals for research. Many financial incentives pave the way for acceptance of protocols that prove deadly and costly. Medical students are even offered incentives through sponsorship by drug companies to prescribe certain drugs as soon as they are able to do so.

The public has accepted the Faustian bargain that his physician has made with the drug companies because the patient believes there is no other choice. He must take ten different prescription drugs if he is over 60. He must have invasive tests. He must have a CT scan with the power of 100 chest X-rays. He must respond to the direct-to-consumer pharmaceutical advertising and ask his doctor to prescribe TV meds, despite the horrific side-effects warnings. The public now receives television messages that appear to be coming from avuncular doctors, but they are really coming from Big Pharma to get your money.

When it comes to choosing between prevention of disease, at least where a condition could be prevented, or treatment of disease, it is advantageous to the allopathic doctor to choose treatment. There is reward in choosing treatment because the drug companies offer incentives to doctors who buy their products. Prevention is more about vitamins and supplements and they are far less lucrative for pharmaceutical companies. There is now a campaign to raise the prices of these natural products that have few, if any, side effects. A prescription may be necessary soon to obtain the vitamins that are now so readily available at reasonable prices. We have the drug companies to thank for this.

For example, if an honest journalist wishes to do an article on the benefits of St. John's Wort for minor depression, he may call several government agencies for a story. If the journalist presents evidence that St. John's Wort is helpful, the FDA and the CDC may *encourage* the journalist to promote *more proven therapies*, such as expensive prescription anti-depressants. They may encourage or even pay the journalist to downplay any merits of St. John's Wort. This is where the drug companies interfere with the public's education about natural remedies. The far-reaching arm of the pharmaceutical company's influence even extends to the falsification of nutrient studies, in order to promote prescription drugs instead. There is currently a systematic program to defame every natural vitamin, supplement, and health food throughout the world.

Corruption is rampant when legislators pay journalists to do a hatchet job on natural preventive remedies, so that the public will buy prescription drugs. Where honest scientists do exist, they have no power to override the corruption. The price they would pay for writing or speaking the truth about the drug company invasion into modern medicine, or for censuring a colleague for cause, is that the doctor or researcher would be alienated, unable to get grants, unable to publish, possibly even unable to work. That rare courageous doctor would have his career destroyed, though his good character would be intact.

The medical environment has become a labyrinth of interlocking corporate, hospital, and governmental boards of directors and advisors, infiltrated by the drug companies. There are even ghost writers who are drug company representatives who write glowing articles about pharmaceuticals, then they are signed by well-known physicians who are paid handsomely for their cooperation, though they may not know all of the adverse side-effects of the drugs they promote. The physicians are paid to give positive reviews of drug company studies; they are paid to endorse chemicals that may harm patients because there is a rush to get the drugs on the market. The most toxic substances are often approved first. Milder alternatives may be ignored for financial reasons.

Drug companies now control the dissemination of continuing education courses to doctors, and there may be some brainwashing going on; ads in medical publications are controlled by drug companies; information given to the FDA to promote is influenced by drug companies; drug companies may pay the FDA to review their studies favorably. Influence is for sale.

There are astronomical profits in cooperating with the drug companies. Drug companies are behind Medicare, so that people remain over-medicated; or they receive the proper medications at higher doses to sell more, with injury or death as a consequence.

Drug companies pay our legislators, our scientists, the NAS. Drug companies have propaganda campaigns launched through the CDC, such as a rush to vaccinate the moment a "bird flu" appears on the horizon. Vaccinate infants, children, teens, adults, elders, each one a potentially lucrative marketing niche, even an opportunity to sell drugs to otherwise healthy people. Why not make these vaccinations mandatory? Force us to pay for possible side effects, "for our own good." Fright tactics are used to petrify the public into rushing to pay for vaccines that may prove debilitating or worse.

All of this is done with a wink and a nod. Not a cent is spent on prevention (except pseudo-prevention through toxic inoculations that do not really prevent disease, and may cause harm); instead, every dollar goes for treatment.

The media, scientists, professors, universities, hospitals, governmental agencies, such as the FDA, the EPA, and the CDC, are all having a banquet at the pharmaceutical table. This is not the way to practice medicine. Every so often, brave physicians like Drs. Graeme Morgan, Robyn Ward, and Michael Barton stand up and tell the truth, about cytotoxic chemotherapy, in this case, as in their article in *Clinical Oncology*, "The Contribution of Cytotoxic Chemotherapy to 5-year Survival in Adult Malignancies." Curative and adjuvant chemotherapy is only 2.1%

effective in America in this study; with no progress in the field over the past 20 years.

There are also a few thousand complementary physicians who are helping patients. Many complementary healthcare providers are denied publication through the intervention of pharmaceutical companies. If they, or their allopathic colleagues, do manage to speak out against corruption in the establishment, they are considered traitors to the medical brotherhood. This is not a scientific community; instead of objectivity and compassion, our medical system is powered by weakness, greed, envy, and fear. There are exceptions, such as Dr. David Graham of the FDA.

Medicine also has many spectacular breakthroughs and modalities for helping people to heal and survive—but let us continue to determine what does not work and request that improvements be made. Let us be honest about the causes of our illnesses. Your average doctor is not telling you that your lifestyle may be making you ill, and that you can do something economical to improve your health, and possibly reduce the need for costly medication he prescribes (never change your medication dosage without your doctor's approval). You are your doctor's "client."

The cumulative daily effects of steaks, colas, pizzas, pollution, computers, cell phones, and pesticides place us in a toxic soup environment. Instead of cleaning this up, many turn to medication for help. Drug companies are paying our legislators, television and radio stations, schools, and news outlets to keep this information from you. You are Big Pharma's "client." BP wants your "account." And they pay the quack busters to attack anyone who tells you the truth about what is really making you sick enough to seek expensive "care" from the number one source of fatalities in America, care that might readily kill you and your loved ones: death by medicine.

References

1. Institute of Medicine, US National Academy of Sciences. November 1999. To Err Is Human: Building a Safer Health System. http://www.iom.edu/Object.File/Master/4/117/ToErr-8pager.pdf (accessed January 25, 2009).

2. Center for Drug Evaluation and Research. U.S. Food and Drug Administration. Preventable Adverse Drug Reactions: A Focus on Drug Interactions. Last updated July 31, 2002. http://www.fda.gov/cder/drug/drugReactions/default.htm#ADRs:%20Prevalence%20and%20Incidence (accessed January 25, 2009).

3. Furberg, C. D., A. A. Levin, P. A. Gross, R. S. Shapiro, and B. L. Strom. 2006. The FDA and drug safety: a proposal for sweeping changes. *Arch Intern Med* 166 (18):1938-42.

4. Gordon S. Antibiotics still prescribed too often, includes interview with expert Dr. Philip

Tierno, originally published by *Health Day News*, November 8, 2005, reprinted by *PharmDaily. com*. http://www.pharmdaily.com/Article/1722/ Antibiotics_Still_Prescribed_Too_Often. html?CategoryID=29 (accessed January 25, 2009).

5. U.S. Centers for Disease Control and Prevention (CDC). It's Time to Get Smart about the Use of Antibiotics: CDC campaign aims to draw attention to the increasing problem of antibiotic resistance, (Press Release), CDC, October 2, 2008. http://www.cdc.gov/media/pressrel/2008/ r081002.htm (accessed January 25, 2009).

6. US National Center for Health Statistics. Deaths: final Data for 2005. *National Vital Statistics Report*, vol. 56, no. 10, April 24, 2008. http://www.cdc.gov/nchs/data/nvsr/nvsr56/ nvsr56_10.pdf (accessed January 24, 2009).

7. National Cancer Institute, US National Institutes of Health. Cancer Statistics (projection for 2008), Surveillance, Epidemiology and End Results (SEER) Stat Fact Sheets, "based on November 2007 SEER data submission, posted to the SEER web site, 2008." http://seer.cancer. gov/statfacts/html/all.html (accessed January 23, 2009).

8. US Senate Finance Committee. Testimony of David J. Graham, MD, MPH, November 18, 2004. http://finance.senate.gov/hearings/ testimony/2004test/111804dgtest.pdf (accessed January 30, 2009).

9. Ibid.

10. Alonso-Zaldivar, R., FDA Called 'Defenseless' Against Unsafe Drugs, *Los Angeles Times*, November 18, 2004. http://www.mcall.com/topic/la-111804vioxx_lat,0,7473253.story (accessed January 31, 2009).

11. US Senate Finance Committee. Testimony of David J. Graham, MD, MPH, November 18, 2004. http://finance.senate.gov/hearings/testimony/2004test/111804dgtest.pdf (accessed January 30, 2009).

12. National Coalition Against Censorship. FDA Suppressed Vioxx Studies Despite Evidence of Serious Health Risks, November 25, 2004. http://www.ncac.org/FDA_Suppressed_Vioxx_Studies (accessed January 30, 2009).

13. Bailey Esq, B., Bad medicine, *Texas Injury Law*, July 27, 2008. http://www.txinjurylawblog.com/tags/drugs-accolate-accutane-arava-1/ (accessed January 30, 2009).

14. Alonso-Zaldivar, R., "FDA Called 'Defenseless' Against Unsafe Drugs," *Los Angeles Times*, November 18, 2004. http://www.mcall.com/topic/la-111804vioxx_lat,0,7473253.story (accessed January 31, 2009).

15. Associated Press. F.D.A. Called 'Defenseless' Against Unsafe Drugs, *New York Times*, 18 November 2004. http://biopsychiatry.com/bigpharma/fda.html (accessed January 31, 2009).

16. *Yale Medicine*. FDA's top safety critic keeps a watchful eye on the public good, Summer 2005.

http://yalemedicine.yale.edu/ym_su05/faces.
html (accessed January 31, 2009).

17. Young, D., Safety Experts Call for Accountability from FDA, Drug Firms. American Society of Health-System Pharmacists, March 23, 2007. http://www.ashp.org/import/News/HealthSystemPharmacyNews/newsarticle.aspx?id=2503 (accessed January 31, 2009).

18. Ibid.

19. Loudon, Manette, interviewer. The FDA Exposed: An Interview With Dr. David Graham, the Vioxx Whistleblower, parts of this interview appear in Gary Null's documentary film, *Prescription for Disaster*, Garynull.com, August 30, 2005, reprinted by *Natural News*. http://www.naturalnews.com/011401.html (accessed January 31, 2009).

20. US Senate Finance Committee. Testimony of David J. Graham, MD, MPH, November 18, 2004. http://finance.senate.gov/hearings/testimony/2004test/111804dgtest.pdf (accessed January 30, 2009).

21. *Yale Medicine*. FDA's top safety critic keeps a watchful eye on the public good, Summer 2005. http://yalemedicine.yale.edu/ym_su05/faces.html (accessed January 31, 2009).

22. Alonso-Zaldivar, R., FDA Called 'Defenseless' Against Unsafe Drugs, *Los Angeles Times*, November 18, 2004. http://www.mcall.com/topic/la-111804vioxx_lat,0,7473253.story (accessed January 31, 2009).

23. Kelly, J. Harsh criticism lobbed at FDA in Senate Vioxx hearing, *Medscape Medical News*, November 23, 2004. http://medgenmed.medscape.com/viewarticle/538021_print (accessed January 31, 2009).

24. Lazarou, J., B. H. Pomeranz, and P. N. Corey. 1998. Incidence of adverse drug reactions in hospitalized patients: a meta-analysis of prospective studies. *JAMA* 279 (15):1200-5.

25. Ibid.

26. Gurwitz, J. H., T. S. Field, J. Avorn, D. McCormick, S. Jain, M. Eckler, M. Benser, A. C. Edmondson, and D. W. Bates. 2000. Incidence and preventability of adverse drug events in nursing homes. *Am J Med* 109 (2):87-94.

27. Center for Drug Evaluation and Research. U.S. Food and Drug Administration. Preventable Adverse Drug Reactions: A Focus on Drug Interactions. Last updated July 31, 2002. http://www.fda.gov/cder/drug/drugReactions/default.htm#ADRs:%20Prevalence%20and%20Incidence (accessed January 25, 2009).

28. Rabin R. Caution about overuse of antibiotics. *Newsday*. September 18, 2003.

29. Available at: http://www.cdc.gov/drugresistance/community/ (Accessed May 22, 2006).

30. Gordon S. Antibiotics still prescribed too often, includes interview with expert Dr. Philip Tierno, originally published by *Health Day News*, November 8, 2005, reprinted by *PharmDaily*.

com. http://www.pharmdaily.com/Article/1722/ Antibiotics_Still_Prescribed_Too_Often. html?CategoryID=29 (accessed January 25, 2009).

31. U.S. Centers for Disease Control and Prevention (CDC). It's Time to Get Smart about the Use of Antibiotics: CDC campaign aims to draw attention to the increasing problem of antibiotic resistance, (Press Release), CDC, October 2, 2008. http://www.cdc.gov/media/pressrel/2008/ r081002.htm (accessed January 25, 2009).

32. Ibid.

33. Available at: http://www.ahrq.gov/data/ hcup/ hcupnet.htm. (accessed May 22, 2006).

34. US Congressional House Subcommittee Oversight Investigation. Cost and Quality of Health Care: Unnecessary Surgery. Washington, DC: Government Printing Office; 1976. Cited in: McClelland GB, Foundation for Chiropractic Education and Research. Testimony to the Department of Veterans Affairs' Chiropractic Advisory Committee. March 25, 2003.

35. http://www.ahrq.gov/data/ hcup/hcupnet.htm. (accessed May 22, 2006).

36. Siu, A. L., F. A. Sonnenberg, W. G. Manning, G. A. Goldberg, E. S. Bloomfield, J. P. Newhouse, and R. H. Brook. 1986. Inappropriate use of hospitals in a randomized trial of health insurance plans. *N Engl J Med* 315 (20):1259-66.

37. Siu, A. L., W. G. Manning, and B. Benjamin. 1990. Patient, provider and hospital characteristics

associated with inappropriate hospitalization. *Am J Public Health* 80 (10):1253-6.

38. Eriksen, B. O., I. S. Kristiansen, E. Nord, J. F. Pape, S. M. Almdahl, A. Hensrud, and S. Jaeger. 1999. The cost of inappropriate admissions: a study of health benefits and resource utilization in a department of internal medicine. *J Intern Med* 246 (4):379-87.

39. National Coalition on Health Care. "Did You Know?" section of home page of NCHC, 2009. http://www.nchc.org/ (accessed January 27, 2009).

40. Weinstein, R. A. 1998. Nosocomial infection update. *Emerg Infect Dis* 4 (3):416-20.

41. Fourth Decennial International Conference on Nosocomial and Healthcare-Associated Infections. Morbidity and Mortality Weekly Report. February 25, 2000, Vol. 49, No. 7, p. 138.

42. Centers for Disease Control and Prevention. Estimates of Healthcare-Associated Infections, last modified May 30, 2007. http://www.cdc.gov/ncidod/dhqp/hai.html (accessed January 24, 2009).

43. Ibid.

44. Klevens, R. Monina DDS, MPH, Jonathan R. Edwards, MS, Chesley L. Richards, Jr., MD, MPH, Teresa C. Horan, MPH, Robert P. Gaynes, MD, Daniel A. Pollock, MD, Denise M. Cardo, MD. Estimating Health Care-Associated Infections and Deaths in U.S. Hospitals, 2002, *Public Health Reports,* Volume 122, March–April 2007.

http://www.cdc.gov/ncidod/dhqp/pdf/hicpac/infections_deaths.pdf (accessed January 27, 2009).

45. US National Center for Health Statistics. Deaths: final Data for 2005. National Vital Statistics Report, vol. 56, no. 10, April 24, 2008. http://www.cdc.gov/nchs/data/nvsr/nvsr56/nvsr56_10.pdf (accessed January 24, 2009).

46. Wyden, Ron Senator, The Healthy Americans Act. "$2.2 trillion currently spent on health care in America today." http://wyden.senate.gov/issues/Legislation/Healthy_Americans_Act.cfm (accessed January 26, 2009).

47. National Coalition on Health Care. Economic Cost Fact Sheets: The Impact of Rising Health Care Costs on the Economy, NCHC, 2009. http://www.nchc.org/facts/economic.shtml (accessed January 27, 2009).

48. Wyden, Ron Senator, The Healthy Americans Act. "$2.2 trillion currently spent on health care in America today." http://wyden.senate.gov/issues/Legislation/Healthy_Americans_Act.cfm (accessed January 26, 2009).

49. Lazarou, J., B. H. Pomeranz, and P. N. Corey. 1998. Incidence of adverse drug reactions in hospitalized patients: a meta- analysis of prospective studies. *JAMA* 279 (15):1200-5.

50. Suh, D. C., B. S. Woodall, S. K. Shin, and E. R. Hermes-De Santis. 2000. Clinical and economic impact of adverse drug reactions in hospitalized patients. *Ann Pharmacother* 34 (12):1373-9.

51. Center for Drug Evaluation and Research. U.S. Food and Drug Administration. Preventable Adverse Drug Reactions: A Focus on Drug Interactions. Last updated July 31, 2002. http://www.fda.gov/cder/drug/drugReactions/default.htm#ADRs:%20Prevalence%20and%20Incidence (accessed January 25, 2009).

52. Institute of Medicine, US National Academy of Sciences. November 1999. To Err Is Human: Building a Safer Health System. http://www.iom.edu/Object.File/Master/4/117/ToErr-8pager.pdf (accessed January 25, 2009).

53. Thomas, E. J., D. M. Studdert, H. R. Burstin, E. J. Orav, T. Zeena, E. J. Williams, K. M. Howard, P. C. Weiler, and T. A. Brennan. 2000. Incidence and types of adverse events and negligent care in Utah and Colorado. *Med Care* 38 (3):261-71.

54. Thomas, E. J., D. M. Studdert, J. P. Newhouse, B. I. Zbar, K. M. Howard, E. J. Williams, and T. A. Brennan. 1999. Costs of medical injuries in Utah and Colorado. *Inquiry* 36 (3):255-64.

55. Xakellis, G. C., R. Frantz, and A. Lewis. 1995. Cost of pressure ulcer prevention in long-term care. *J Am Geriatr Soc* 43 (5):496-501.

56. Barczak, C. A., R. I. Barnett, E. J. Childs, and L. M. Bosley. 1997. Fourth national pressure ulcer prevalence survey. *Adv Wound Care* 10 (4):18-26.

57. Centers for Disease Control and Prevention. Estimates of Healthcare-Associated Infections, last modified May 30, 2007. http://www.cdc.

gov/ncidod/dhqp/hai.html (accessed January 24, 2009).

58. Weinstein, R. A. 1998. Nosocomial infection update. *Emerg Infect Dis* 4 (3):416-20.

59. Fourth Decennial International Conference on Nosocomial and Healthcare-Associated Infections. Morbidity and Mortality Weekly Report. February 25, 2000, Vol. 49, No. 7, p. 138.

60. Available at: http://www.cmwf.org/programs/ elders/burger_mal_386.asp. (accessed May 22, 2006).

61. Starfield, B. 2000. Is US health really the best in the world? *JAMA* 284 (4):483-5.

62. Starfield, B. 2000. Deficiencies in US medical care. *JAMA* 284 (17):2184-5.

63. Weingart, S. N., L. Wilson R. Mc, R. W. Gibberd, and B. Harrison. 2000. Epidemiology of medical error. *West J Med* 172 (6):390-3.

64. Siu, A. L., W. G. Manning, and B. Benjamin. 1990. Patient, provider and hospital characteristics associated with inappropriate hospitalization. *Am J Public Health* 80 (10):1253-6.

65. Thomas, E. J., D. M. Studdert, J. P. Newhouse, B. I. Zbar, K. M. Howard, E. J. Williams, and T. A. Brennan. 1999. Costs of medical injuries in Utah and Colorado. *Inquiry* 36 (3):255-64.

66. Available at: http://www.ahrq.gov/news/ ress/ pr2003/injurypr.htm. (Accessed May 22, 2006).

67. National Coalition on Health Care. Health Insurance Costs: Facts on the Cost of Health Insurance and Health Care, NCHC, 2009. http://

www.nchc.org/facts/cost.shtml (accessed January 28, 2009).

68. National Coalition on Health Care. "Did You Know?" section of home page of NCHC, 2009. http://www.nchc.org/ (accessed January 27, 2009).

69. National Coalition on Health Care. Health Insurance Costs: Facts on the Cost of Health Insurance and Health Care, NCHC, 2009. http://www.nchc.org/facts/cost.shtml (accessed January 28, 2009).

70. National Coalition on Health Care. "Did You Know?" section of home page of NCHC, 2009. http://www.nchc.org/ (accessed January 27, 2009).

71. Lazarou, J., B. H. Pomeranz, and P. N. Corey. 1998. Incidence of adverse drug reactions in hospitalized patients: a meta-analysis of prospective studies. *JAMA* 279 (15):1200-5.

72. National Patient Safety Foundation. Nationwide poll on patient safety: 100 million Americans see medical mistakes directly touching them [press release]. McLean, VA: October 9, 1997.

73. Leape, L. L. 1994. Error in medicine. *JAMA* 272 (23):1851-7.

74. National Patient Safety Foundation. Nationwide poll on patient safety: 100 million Americans see medical mistakes directly touching them [press release]. McLean, VA: October 9, 1997.

75. Xakellis, G. C., R. Frantz, and A. Lewis. 1995. Cost of pressure ulcer prevention in long-term care. *J Am Geriatr Soc* 43 (5):496-501.

76. Barczak, C. A., R. I. Barnett, E. J. Childs, and L. M. Bosley. 1997. Fourth national pressure

ulcer prevalence survey. *Adv Wound Care* 10 (4):18-26.

77. Centers for Disease Control and Prevention. Estimates of Healthcare-Associated Infections, last modified May 30, 2007. http://www.cdc.gov/ncidod/dhqp/hai.html (accessed January 24, 2009).

78. Weinstein, R. A. 1998. Nosocomial infection update. *Emerg Infect Dis* 4 (3):416-20.

79. Fourth Decennial International Conference on Nosocomial and Healthcare-Associated Infections. Morbidity and Mortality Weekly Report. February 25, 2000, Vol. 49, No. 7, p. 138.

80. Available at: http://www.cmwf.org/programs/elders/burger_mal_386.asp. (accessed May 22, 2006).

81. Starfield, B. 2000. Is US health really the best in the world? *JAMA* 284 (4):483-5.

82. Starfield, B. 2000. Deficiencies in US medical care. *JAMA* 284 (17):2184-5.

83. Weingart, S. N., L. Wilson R. Mc, R. W. Gibberd, and B. Harrison. 2000. Epidemiology of medical error. *West J Med* 172 (6):390-3.

84. Available at: http://www.ahrq.gov/data/ hcup/hcupnet.htm. (accessed May 22, 2006).

85. Available at: http://www.ahrq.gov/news/ ress/pr2003/injurypr.htm. (Accessed May 22, 2006).

86. Peck, P. Patient safety requires fundamental changes to medical systems. *Medscape Medical News*, 6 May 2004. http://www.medscape.com/viewarticle/475217 (accessed January 28, 2009).

87. Altman, LK. Even the elite hospitals aren't immune to errors. *New York Times*, 23 February 2003. http://query.nytimes.com/gst/fullpage.html?res=9C0DE3D9113DF930A15751C0A9659C8B63&n=Top/Reference/Times%20Topics/People/S/Santillan,%20Jesica&scp=1&sq=Altman%20LK.%20Even%20the%20elite%20hospitals%20aren%E2%80%99t%20immune%20to%20errors.%20New%20York%20Times,%2023%20February%202003&st=cse (accessed January 28, 2009).

88. Lazarou, J., B. H. Pomeranz, and P. N. Corey. 1998. Incidence of adverse drug reactions in hospitalized patients: a meta-analysis of prospective studies. *JAMA* 279 (15):1200-5.

89. Weinstein, R. A. 1998. Nosocomial infection update. *Emerg Infect Dis* 4 (3):416-20.

90. Leape, L. L. 1994. Error in medicine. *JAMA* 272 (23):1851-7.

91. LaPointe, N. M., and J. G. Jollis. 2003. Medication errors in hospitalized cardiovascular patients. *Arch Intern Med* 163 (12):1461-6.

92. Lazarou, J., B. H. Pomeranz, and P. N. Corey. 1998. Incidence of adverse drug reactions in hospitalized patients: a meta-analysis of prospective studies. *JAMA* 279 (15):1200-5.

93. Institute of Medicine, US National Academy of Sciences. November 1999. To Err Is Human: Building a Safer Health System. http://www.iom.edu/Object.File/Master/4/117/ToErr-8pager.pdf (accessed January 25, 2009).

94. Thomas, E. J., D. M. Studdert, H. R. Burstin, E. J. Orav, T. Zeena, E. J. Williams, K. M. Howard, P. C. Weiler, and T. A. Brennan. 2000. Incidence and types of adverse events and negligent care in Utah and Colorado. *Med Care* 38 (3):261-71.

95. Thomas, E. J., D. M. Studdert, J. P. Newhouse, B. I. Zbar, K. M. Howard, E. J. Williams, and T. A. Brennan. 1999. Costs of medical injuries in Utah and Colorado. *Inquiry* 36 (3):255-64.

96. Xakellis, G. C., R. Frantz, and A. Lewis. 1995. Cost of pressure ulcer prevention in long-term care. *J Am Geriatr Soc* 43 (5):496-501.

97. Barczak, C. A., R. I. Barnett, E. J. Childs, and L. M. Bosley. 1997. Fourth national pressure ulcer prevalence survey. *Adv Wound Care* 10 (4):18-26.

98. Centers for Disease Control and Prevention. Estimates of Healthcare-Associated Infections, last modified May 30, 2007. http://www.cdc.gov/ncidod/dhqp/hai.html (accessed January 24, 2009).

99. Weinstein, R. A. 1998. Nosocomial infection update. *Emerg Infect Dis* 4 (3):416-20.

100. Fourth Decennial International Conference on Nosocomial and Healthcare-Associated Infections. Morbidity and Mortality Weekly Report. February 25, 2000, Vol. 49, No. 7, p. 138.

101. Available at: http://www.cmwf.org/programs/elders/burger_mal_386.asp. (accessed May 22, 2006).

102. Starfield, B. 2000. Is US health really the best in the world? *JAMA* 284 (4):483-5.

103. Starfield, B. 2000. Deficiencies in US medical care. *JAMA* 284 (17):2184-5.

104. Weingart, S. N., L. Wilson R. Mc, R. W. Gibberd, and B. Harrison. 2000. Epidemiology of medical error. *West J Med* 172 (6):390-3.

105. Available at: http://www.ahrq.gov/data/ hcup/ hcupnet.htm. (accessed May 22, 2006).

106. Available at: http://www.ahrq.gov/news/ ress/ pr2003/injurypr.htm. (Accessed May 22, 2006).

107. http://www.ahrq.gov/data/ hcup/hcupnet.htm. (accessed May 22, 2006).

108. Siu, A. L., F. A. Sonnenberg, W. G. Manning, G. A. Goldberg, E. S. Bloomfield, J. P. Newhouse, and R. H. Brook. 1986. Inappropriate use of hospitals in a randomized trial of health insurance plans. *N Engl J Med* 315 (20):1259-66.

109. Siu, A. L., W. G. Manning, and B. Benjamin. 1990. Patient, provider and hospital characteristics associated with inappropriate hospitalization. *Am J Public Health* 80 (10):1253-6.

110. Eriksen, B. O., I. S. Kristiansen, E. Nord, J. F. Pape, S. M. Almdahl, A. Hensrud, and S. Jaeger. 1999. The cost of inappropriate admissions: a study of health benefits and resource utilization in a department of internal medicine. *J Intern Med* 246 (4):379-87.

111. Available at: http://www.ahrq.gov/data/ hcup/ hcupnet.htm. (accessed May 22, 2006).

112. The Society of Actuaries Health Benefit Systems Practice Advancement Committee. The Troubled Healthcare System in the US. September 13, 2003.

Available at: http://www.soa.org/sections/
troubled_healthcare.pdf. (accessed December
18, 2003).

113. National Coalition on Health Care. Health Insurance Costs: Facts on the Cost of Health Insurance and Health Care, NCHC, 2009. http://
www.nchc.org/facts/cost.shtml (accessed January 28, 2009).

114. Shafrin, J., Ph.D. candidate in Economics at UC,
U.S. spends $700 billion on unnecessary medical
tests, *Healthcare Economist*, November 7, 2008.
http://healthcare-economist.com/2008/11/07/
us-spends-700-billion-on-unnecessary-medical-
tests/ (accessed January 28, 2009).

115. Berenson, A. and R. Abelson, The Evidence Gap:
Weighing the Costs of a CT Scan's Look Inside the
Heart, *New York Times*, June 29, 2008. http://www.
nytimes.com/2008/06/29/business/29scan.
html?_r=1&ei=5087&em=&en=fe03ca7fee
00b38f&ex=1214971200&adxnnl=1&adxn
nlx=1214838413-Ndu72SwNDujyHmtVwDa+AA
(accessed January 28, 2009).

116. National Coalition for Health Care. 2009. Facts
on Health Insurance Coverage. http://www.
nchc.org/facts/coverage.shtml (accessed January 31, 2009).

117. Ibid.

118. Families USA. Wrong Direction: One Out of Three
Americans are Uninsured. September 2007. http://
familiesusa.org/assets/pdfs/wrong-direction.pdf
(accessed January 31, 2009).

119. National Coalition for Health Care. 2009. Facts on Health Insurance Coverage. http://www.nchc.org/facts/coverage.shtml (accessed January 31, 2009).

120. Ibid.

121. Alonso-Zaldivar, R. Getting married for health insurance, *Los Angeles Times,* April 29, 2008. http://articles.latimes.com/2008/apr/29/nation/na-health29 (accessed January 31, 2009).

122. Alonso-Zaldivar, R. Getting married for health insurance, *Los Angeles Times,* April 29, 2008. http://articles.latimes.com/2008/apr/29/nation/na-health29 (accessed January 31, 2009).

123. Institute of Medicine. Care Without Coverage: Too Little, Too Late. May 21, 2002. A Shared Destiny: Community Effects of Uninsurance. March 6, 2003.

124. US Department of Health and Human Services and US Department of Justice. Health Care Fraud and Abuse Control Program Annual Report for FY 1998. April 1999. Health Care Fraud and Abuse Control Program Annual Report for FY 2001. April 2002.

125. Leape, L. L. 1994. Error in medicine. *JAMA* 272 (23):1851-7.

126. Bates, D. W., D. J. Cullen, N. Laird, L. A. Petersen, S. D. Small, D. Servi, G. Laffel, B. J. Sweitzer, B. F. Shea, R. Hallisey, and et al. 1995. Incidence of adverse drug events and potential adverse drug events. Implications for prevention. ADE Prevention Study Group. *JAMA* 274 (1):29-34.

127. Vincent, C., N. Stanhope and M. Crowley-Murphy. Reasons for not reporting adverse incidents: an empirical study. J Eval Clin Pract. 1999 Feb;5(1):13-21.

128. Bates, DW. Drugs and adverse drug reactions: how worried should we be? *JAMA*. 1998 Apr 15;279(15):1216-7.

129. Dickinson, JG. FDA seeks to double effort on confusing drug names. Dickinson's FDA Review. 2000 Mar;7(3):13-4.

130. Leape, L. L. 1994. Error in medicine. *JAMA* 272 (23):1851-7.

131. Campbell, E. G., J. S. Weissman, B. Clarridge, R. Yucel, N. Causino, and D. Blumenthal. 2003. Characteristics of medical school faculty members serving on institutional review boards: results of a national survey. *Acad Med* 78 (8):831-6.

132. HealthDayNews. Possible conflict of interest within medical profession. August 15, 2003.

133. Harris, G. F.D.A. Limits Role of Advisers Tied to Industry, *The New York Times*, March 22, 2007. http://www.nytimes.com/2007/03/22/washington/22fda.html (accessed January 26, 2009).

134. Leape, L. L. 1994. Error in medicine. *JAMA* 272 (23):1851-7.

135. Brennan, T. A., L. L. Leape, N. M. Laird, L. Hebert, A. R. Localio, A. G. Lawthers, J. P. Newhouse, P. C. Weiler, and H. H. Hiatt. 1991. Incidence of adverse events and negligence in hospitalized

patients. Results of the Harvard Medical Practice Study I. *N Engl J Med* 324 (6):370-6.

136. Bates, D. W., D. J. Cullen, N. Laird, L. A. Petersen, S. D. Small, D. Servi, G. Laffel, B. J. Sweitzer, B. F. Shea, R. Hallisey, and et al. 1995. Incidence of adverse drug events and potential adverse drug events. Implications for prevention. ADE Prevention Study Group. *JAMA* 274 (1):29-34.

137. National Patient Safety Foundation. Nationwide poll on patient safety: 100 million Americans see medical mistakes directly touching them [press release]. McLean, VA: October 9, 1997.

138. Leape, L. L. 1994. Error in medicine. *JAMA* 272 (23):1851-7.

139. Kotulak, R. Doctors' haste seen hurting patient: study says the push for quick treatment detracts from care. *Chicago Tribune online edition*, 10 May 2005. http://www.chicagotribune. com/features/health/ (no longer available here); available at Committee for Justice for All: Patient Safety and Doctor Discipline, CJA President Attorney Peter I. Fallk, Dr. Persell quote is on website. http://www.saynotocaps. org/patientsafety.shtml (accessed January 28, 2009).

140. Leape, L. L. 1994. Error in medicine. *JAMA* 272 (23):1851-7.

141. Vincent, C., N. Stanhope and M. Crowley-Murphy. Reasons for not reporting adverse incidents: an empirical study. J Eval Clin Pract. 1999 Feb;5(1):13-21.

142. Wald, H., Shojania, K.G. Incident reporting. In: Shojania, K.G., Duncan, B.W., McDonald, K.M., et al, eds. Making Health Care Safer: A Critical Analysis of Patient Safety Practices. Rockville, MD: Agency for Healthcare Research and Quality; 2001:chapter 4. Evidence Report/Technology Assessment No. 43. AHRQ publication 01-E058.

143. Grinfeld, M.J. The debate over medical error reporting. *Psychiatric Times*. April 2000.

144. Ibid.

145. King, G. III, A. Hermodson. 2000. Peer reporting of coworker wrongdoing: a qualitative analysis of observer attitudes in the decision to report versus not report unethical behavior. *Journal of Applied Communication Research* (28), 309-29.

146. Stenson, J. Few residents report medical errors, survey finds. Reuters Health. February 21, 2003.

147. Agency for Healthcare Research and Quality. Underreporting of medical errors affecting children is a significant problem, particularly among physicians," [federal] http://www.ahrq.gov/research/dec04/1204RA7.htm (accessed January 29, 2009).

148. Taylor, J.A., D. Brownstein, D.A. Christakis, S. Blackburn, T.P. Strandjord, E.J. Klein and J. Shafii. Use of incident reports by physicians and nurses to document medical errors in pediatric patients. *Pediatrics* 114(3):Sept 2004, pp. 729-735; http://pediatrics.aappublications.org/cgi/content/abstract/114/3/729 (accessed January 29, 2009).

149. Indiana University School of Medicine, WFYI 90.1 FM radio program, host Jeremy Shere, "Doctors Don't Report Medical Errors," interview with Lauris Kaldjian, M.D., Ph.D., Director of Bioethics Program of U. Iowa, to discuss his report on medical errors, which appears in the Jan. 14, 2008 issue of *Archives of Internal Medicine,* on "Sound Medicine Checkup," aired on February 17, 2008. http://soundmedicine.iu.edu/segment. php4?seg=1522 (accessed January 28, 2009).

150. Blendon, R. J., C. Schoen, C. M. DesRoches, R. Osborn, K. L. Scoles, and K. Zapert. 2002. Inequities in health care: a five-country survey. *Health Aff (Millwood)* 21 (3):182-91.

151. Harvard School of Public Health. Survey by Henry J. Kaiser Family Foundation, Methodology: Fieldwork conducted by ICR - International Communications Research, April 11-June 11, 2002.

152. Patient Safety and Quality Improvement Act of 2005. Pub L 109-41. http://frwebgate.access. gpo.gov/cgi-bin/getdoc.cgi?dbname=109_cong_ public_laws&docid=f:publ041.109.pdf (accessed January 29, 2009).

153. *The Patient Safety and Quality Improvement Act of 2005.* Overview, June 2008. Agency for Healthcare Research and Quality, Rockville, MD. http:// www.ahrq.gov/qual/psoact.htm (accessed January 29, 2009).

154. Lazarou, J., B. H. Pomeranz, and P. N. Corey. 1998. Incidence of adverse drug reactions in

hospitalized patients: a meta-analysis of prospective studies. *JAMA* 279 (15):1200-5.

155. Tauber, Michelle. The Quaid Twins 'Fighting for Their Lives': Dennis and Kimberly Quaid Keep Vigil as Their Newborns Struggle to Survive a Devastating Hospital Error That Resulted in an Overdose of Blood Thinner, *People* Magazine, vol.68, no.24, December 10, 2007. http://www.people. com/people/archive/article/0,,20170884,00. html (accessed January 29, 2009).

156. ScienceDaily. Largest Ever Prospective Medical Study Shows Epidurals And Spinal Anesthetics Are Safer Than Previously Reported [in Britain], *ScienceDaily, January 16, 2009.* http://www.science-daily.com/releases/2009/01/090113074445. htm *(accessed February 1, 2009).*

157. FAQ's: Anesthesia and Brain Monitoring: What are the risks of anesthesia? *Aspect Medical Systems*, 2009. http://www.aspectmedical.com/patients/ anesthesia-risks.mspx (accessed February 1, 2009).

158. Bond, C. A., C. L. Raehl, and T. Franke. 2002. Clinical pharmacy services, hospital pharmacy staffing, and medication errors in United States hospitals. *Pharmacotherapy* 22 (2):134-47.

159. Barker, K. N., E. A. Flynn, G. A. Pepper, D. W. Bates, and R. L. Mikeal. 2002. Medication errors observed in 36 health care facilities. *Arch Intern Med* 162 (16):1897-903.

160. LaPointe, N. M., and J. G. Jollis. 2003. Medication errors in hospitalized cardiovascular patients. *Arch Intern Med* 163 (12):1461-6.

161. Lazarou, J., B. H. Pomeranz, and P. N. Corey. 1998. Incidence of adverse drug reactions in hospitalized patients: a meta-analysis of prospective studies. *JAMA* 279 (15):1200-5.

162. Ibid.

163. Available at: www.msnbc.com/news/ 937302. asp?cp1=1. (accessed May 22, 2006).

164. Lasser, K. E., P. D. Allen, S. J. Woolhandler, D. U. Himmelstein, S. M. Wolfe, and D. H. Bor. 2002. Timing of new black box warnings and withdrawals for prescription medications. *JAMA* 287 (17):2215-20.

165. Lazarou, J., B. H. Pomeranz, and P. N. Corey. 1998. Incidence of adverse drug reactions in hospitalized patients: a meta-analysis of prospective studies. *JAMA* 279 (15):1200-5.

166. Gandhi, T. K., S. N. Weingart, J. Borus, A. C. Seger, J. Peterson, E. Burdick, D. L. Seger, K. Shu, F. Federico, L. L. Leape, and D. W. Bates. 2003. Adverse drug events in ambulatory care. *N Engl J Med* 348 (16):1556-64.

167. Reuters. Medication side effects strike 1 in 4. April 17, 2003.

168. Rosen, M. Top 20 big pharmas represent majority of world pharma market. *Wisconsin Technology Network*; data drawn from *Pharmaceutial Executive*, May 2005 (IMS Health data). http://wistechnology.com/article.php?id=1903 (accessed January 29, 2009).

169. Gilman, A.G., T.W. Rall, A.S. Nies and P. Taylor. Goodman and Gilman's The Pharma-cological

Basis of Therapeutics. (New York: Pergamon Press; 1996).

170. Kolata, G. New York Times News Service. Who cares when our drugs fail? *San Diego Union-Tribune*, October 15, 1997:E-1,5.

171. Melmon, K.L., H.F. Morrelli, B.B. Hoffman and D.W. Nierenberg, eds. *Melmon and Morrelli's Clinical Pharmacology: Basic Principles in Therapeutics*. 3rd ed. (New York: McGraw-Hill, Inc., 1992).

172. Cullen, D. J., D. W. Bates, S. D. Small, J. B. Cooper, A. R. Nemeskal, and L. L. Leape. 1995. The incident reporting system does not detect adverse drug events: a problem for quality improvement. *Jt Comm J Qual Improv* 21 (10):541-8.

173. Bates, DW. Drugs and advrse drug reactions: how worried should we be? *JAMA*. 1998 Apr 15;279(15):1216-7.

174. Dickinson, JG. FDA seeks to double effort on confusing drug names. Dickinson's FDA Review. 2000 Mar;7(3):13-4.

175. Cohen, J.S. *Overdose: The Case Against the Drug Companies*. (New York: Tarcher-Putnum, 2001).

176. Vastag, B. 2001. Pay attention: ritalin acts much like cocaine. *JAMA* 286 (8):905-6.

177. Bailey Esq, B., Bad medicine, *Texas Injury Law*, July 27, 2008. http://www.txinjurylawblog.com/tags/drugs-accolate-accutane-arava-1/ (accessed January 30, 2009).

178. Rosenthal, M. B., E. R. Berndt, J. M. Donohue, R. G. Frank, and A. M. Epstein. 2002. Promotion of

prescription drugs to consumers. *N Engl J Med* 346 (7):498-505.

179. Wolfe, S. M. 2002. Direct-to-consumer advertising—education or emotion promotion? *N Engl J Med* 346 (7):524-6.

180. Ibid.

181. Testimony and official submissions: PhRMA Chief Medical Officer testifies on DTC advertising, *The Pharmaceutical Research and Manufacturers of America (PhRMA)*, 29 September 2005. http://www.phrma.org/publications/testimony_and_official_submissions/phrma_chief_medical_officer_testifies_on_direct-to-consumer_advertising/ (accessed January 29, 2009).

182. Weissman, J. S., D. Blumenthal, A. J. Silk, M. Newman, K. Zapert, R. Leitman, and S. Feibelmann. 2004. Physicians report on patient encounters involving direct-to-consumer advertising. *Health Aff (Millwood)* Suppl Web Exclusives:W4-219-33. http://content.healthaffairs.org/cgi/content/abstract/hlthaff.w4.219v1 (accessed January 29, 2009).

183. Kaiser Family Foundation, Menlo Park, CA. *Prescription Drug Trends*, Fact Sheet, June 2006." http://www.kff.org/rxdrugs/upload/3057-05.pdf (accessed January 29, 2009).

184. Loudon, Manette, interviewer. "The FDA Exposed: An Interview With Dr. David Graham, the Vioxx Whistleblower," parts of this interview appear in Gary Null's documentary film, "Prescription for Disaster," Garynull.com, August 30,

2005, reprinted by *Natural News*.http://www. naturalnews.com/011401.html (accessed January 31, 2009).

185. US General Accounting Office. Report to the Chairman, Subcommittee on Human Resources and Intergovernmental Relations, Committee on Government Operations, House of Representatives: FDA Drug Review Postapproval Risks 1976-85. Washington, DC: US General Accounting Office; 1990:3.

186. Available at: www.msnbc.com/news/ 937302. asp?cp1=1. (accessed May 22, 2006).

187. Suh, D. C., B. S. Woodall, S. K. Shin, and E. R. Hermes-De Santis. 2000. Clinical and economic impact of adverse drug reactions in hospitalized patients. *Ann Pharmacother* 34 (12):1373-9.

188. Ohlsen, K., T. Ternes, G. Werner, U. Wallner, D. Loffler, W. Ziebuhr, W. Witte, and J. Hacker. 2003. Impact of antibiotics on conjugational resistance gene transfer in Staphylococcus aureus in sewage. *Environ Microbiol* 5 (8):711-6.

189. Pawlowski, S., T. Ternes, M. Bonerz, T. Kluczka, B. van der Burg, H. Nau, L. Erdinger, and T. Braunbeck. 2003. Combined in situ and in vitro assessment of the estrogenic activity of sewage and surface water samples. *Toxicol Sci* 75 (1):57-65.

190. Ternes, T. A., J. Stuber, N. Herrmann, D. McDowell, A. Ried, M. Kampmann, and B. Teiser. 2003. Ozonation: a tool for removal of pharmaceuticals, contrast media and musk fragrances from wastewater? *Water Res* 37 (8):1976-82.

191. Ternes, T. A., M. Meisenheimer, D. McDowell, F. Sacher, H. J. Brauch, B. Haist-Gulde, G. Preuss, U. Wilme, and N. Zulei-Seibert. 2002. Removal of pharmaceuticals during drinking water treatment. *Environ Sci Technol* 36 (17):3855-63.

192. Ternes, T., M. Bonerz, and T. Schmidt. 2001. Determination of neutral pharmaceuticals in wastewater and rivers by liquid chromatography-electrospray tandem mass spectrometry. *J Chromatogr A* 938 (1-2):175-85.

193. Golet, E. M., A. C. Alder, A. Hartmann, T. A. Ternes, and W. Giger. 2001. Trace determination of fluoroquinolone antibacterial agents in urban wastewater by solid-phase extraction and liquid chromatography with fluorescence detection. *Anal Chem* 73 (15):3632-8.

194. Daughton, C. G., and T. A. Ternes. 1999. Pharmaceuticals and personal care products in the environment: agents of subtle change? *Environ Health Perspect* 107 Suppl 6:907-38.

195. Hirsch, R., T. Ternes, K. Haberer, and K. L. Kratz. 1999. Occurrence of antibiotics in the aquatic environment. *Sci Total Environ* 225 (1-2):109-18.

196. Ternes, T. A., M. Stumpf, J. Mueller, K. Haberer, R. D. Wilken, and M. Servos. 1999. Behavior and occurrence of estrogens in municipal sewage treatment plants—I. Investigations in Germany, Canada and Brazil. *Sci Total Environ* 225 (1-2):81-90.

197. Kaufman, M. Drugmaker to pay FDA $500 million. Manufacturing problems found at Schering-Plough. *Washington Post*. May 18, 2002:A01.

198. Agger, W. A. 2002. Antibiotic resistance: unnatural selection in the office and on the farm. *WMJ* 101 (5):12-3.

199. Nash, D. R., J. Harman, E. R. Wald, and K. J. Kelleher. 2002. Antibiotic prescribing by primary care physicians for children with upper respiratory tract infections. *Arch Pediatr Adolesc Med* 156 (11):1114-9.

200. Schindler, C., J. Krappweis, I. Morgenstern, and W. Kirch. 2003. Prescriptions of systemic antibiotics for children in Germany aged between 0 and 6 years. *Pharmacoepidemiol Drug Saf* 12 (2):113-20.

201. Finkelstein, J. A., C. Stille, J. Nordin, R. Davis, M. A. Raebel, D. Roblin, A. S. Go, D. Smith, C. C. Johnson, K. Kleinman, K. A. Chan, and R. Platt. 2003. Reduction in antibiotic use among US children, 1996-2000. *Pediatrics* 112 (3 Pt 1):620-7.

202. Linder, J. A., and R. S. Stafford. 2001. Antibiotic treatment of adults with sore throat by community primary care physicians: a national survey, 1989-1999. *JAMA* 286 (10):1181-6.

203. Available at: http://www.cdc.gov/drugresistance/community/. (accessed May 22, 2006).

204. Rabin R. Caution about overuse of antibiotics. *Newsday*. September 18, 2003.

205. Available at: http://www.cdc.gov/drugresistance/community/ (Accessed May 22, 2006).

206. Weinstein, R. A. 1998. Nosocomial infection update. *Emerg Infect Dis* 4 (3):416-20.

207. Available at: http://www.health.state.ok.us/ program/cdd/ar/. (accessed May 22, 2006).

208. Available at: www.bayer.com/social-responsibility/ health-projects/libra-initiative/page1193.htm. (accessed May 22, 2006).

209. Agency for Healthcare Research and Quality, Rockville, MD. *Health Care-Associated Infections*. AHRQ Publication No. 08-M068, August 2008. http://www.ahrq.gov/qual/haiflyer.htm (accessed February 1, 2009).

210. Coste, J., C. Hanotin, and E. Leutenegger. 1995. [Prescription of non-steroidal anti-inflammatory agents and risk of iatrogenic adverse effects: a survey of 1072 French general practitioners]. *Therapie* 50 (3):265-70.

211. Kouyanou, K., C. E. Pither, and S. Wessely. 1997. Iatrogenic factors and chronic pain. *Psychosom Med* 59 (6):597-604.

212. Hochman, JS. NSAID deaths. NSAIDs in the news, Our Chronic Pain Mission, 2003. http:// www.cpmission.com/main/NSAIDSs2.html (accessed January 29, 2009).

213. Li, D. K., L. Liu, and R. Odouli. 2003. Exposure to non-steroidal anti-inflammatory drugs during pregnancy and risk of miscarriage: population based cohort study. *BMJ* 327 (7411):368. http:// www.bmj.com/cgi/content/full/327/7411/368 (accessed January 29, 2009).

214. *Wilmington Star News* (NC) Study: Painkillers can increase miscarriage risk. Wire article. 16 August 2003, NSAIDS in the news. http://www.

cpmission.com/main/NSAIDs2.html; accessed January 29, 2009.

215. Merck. Merck Announces Voluntary Worldwide Withdrawal of VIOXX, press release, September 30, 2004. http://www.merck.com/newsroom/vioxx_withdrawal/pdf/vioxx_press_release_final.pdfhttp://www.merck.com/newsroom/vioxx_withdrawal/pdf/vioxx_press_release_final.pdf (accessed January 29, 2009).

216. Merck. Merck Announces Voluntary Worldwide Withdrawal of VIOXX, press release, September 30, 2004. http://www.merck.com/newsroom/vioxx_withdrawal/pdf/vioxx_press_release_final.pdfhttp://www.merck.com/newsroom/vioxx_withdrawal/pdf/vioxx_press_release_final.pdf (accessed January 29, 2009).

217. Vioxx: Frequently Asked Questions, What is Vioxx? http://vioxxlawsuit.lawinfo.com/frequently-asked-vioxx-questions.html (accessed January 29, 2009); originally at http://www.nlm.nih.gov/medlineplus/druginfo/medmaster/a699046.html.

218. Juni, P., L. Nartey, S. Reichenbach, R. Sterchi, P. A. Dieppe, and M. Egger. 2004. Risk of cardiovascular events and rofecoxib: cumulative meta-analysis. *Lancet* 364 (9450):2021-9. http://www.thelancet.com/journals/lancet/article/PIIS0140-6736(04)17514-4/fulltext (accessed January 29, 2009).

219. Laurance, J. and S. Foley. Safety review ordered into popular painkillers, The Independent, 22 October

2004. http://www.independent.co.uk/life-style/ health-and-wellbeing/health-news/safety-review-ordered-into-popular-painkillers-544615.html (accessed January 29, 2009).

220. US Senate Finance Committee. Testimony of David J. Graham, MD, MPH, November 18, 2004. http://finance.senate.gov/hearings/ testimony/2004test/111804dgtest.pdf (accessed January 30, 2009).

221. Sardi, Bill. Just How Many Americans Did Vioxx Kill? Lew Rockwell website, former congressional chief of staff to Ron Paul, M.D., April 21, 2006. http://www.lewrockwell.com/sardi/ sardi53.html (accessed January 29, 2009).

222. US Senate Finance Committee. Testimony of David J. Graham, MD, MPH, November 18, 2004. http://finance.senate.gov/hearings/ testimony/2004test/111804dgtest.pdf (accessed January 30, 2009).

223. Abel, U. 1992. Chemotherapy of advanced epithelial cancer—a critical review. *Biomed Pharmacother* 46 (10):439-52.

224. Schulman, K. A., E. A. Stadtmauer, S. D. Reed, H. A. Glick, L. J. Goldstein, J. M. Pines, J. A. Jackman, S. Suzuki, M. J. Styler, P. A. Crilley, T. R. Klumpp, K. F. Mangan, and J. H. Glick. 2003. Economic analysis of conventional-dose chemotherapy compared with high-dose chemotherapy plus autologous hematopoietic stem-cell transplantation for metastatic breast cancer. *Bone Marrow Transplant* 31 (3):205-10.

225. Hassett, M. J., A. J. O'Malley, J. R. Pakes, J. P. Newhouse, and C. C. Earle. 2006. Frequency and cost of chemotherapy-related serious adverse effects in a population sample of women with breast cancer. *J Natl Cancer Inst* 98 (16):1108-17.

226. Ibid.

227. Ibid.

228. Morgan, G., R. Ward, and M. Barton. 2004. The contribution of cytotoxic chemotherapy to 5-year survival in adult malignancies. *Clin Oncol (R Coll Radiol)* 16 (8):549-60. Reports that "The overall contribution of curative and adjuvant cytotoxic chemotherapy to 5-year survival in adults was estimated to be...2.1%" in America.

229. US Congressional House Subcommittee Oversight Investigation. Cost and Quality of Health Care: Unnecessary Surgery. Washington, DC: Government Printing Office; 1976. Cited in: McClelland GB, Foundation for Chiropractic Education and Research. Testimony to the Department of Veterans Affairs' Chiropractic Advisory Committee. March 25, 2003.

230. Leape LL. Unnecessary surgery. Health Serv Res. 1989 Aug;24(3):351-407.

231. Available at: http://www.ahrq.gov/data/ hcup/ hcupnet.htm. (accessed May 22, 2006).

232. US Congressional House Subcommittee Oversight Investigation. Cost and Quality of Health Care: Unnecessary Surgery. Washington, DC: Government Printing Office; 1976. Cited in: McClelland GB, Foundation for Chiropractic Education and

Research. Testimony to the Department of Veterans Affairs' Chiropractic Advisory Committee. March 25, 2003.

233. Leape LL. Unnecessary surgery. Health Serv Res. 1989 Aug; 24(3):351-407.

234. US Congressional House Subcommittee Oversight Investigation. Cost and Quality of Health Care: Unnecessary Surgery. Washington, DC: Government Printing Office; 1976. Cited in: McClelland GB, Foundation for Chiropractic Education and Research. Testimony to the Department of Veterans Affairs' Chiropractic Advisory Committee. March 25, 2003.

235. Available at: http://www.ahrq.gov/data/ hcup/ hcupnet.htm. (accessed May 22, 2006).

236. McClelland GB, Foundation for Chiropractic Education and Research. Testimony to the Department of Veterans Affairs' Chiropractic Advisory Committee. March 25, 2003.

237. Coile, R. C., Jr. 2003. Internet-driven surgery. *Russ Coiles Health Trends* 15 (8):2-4.

238. Guarner, V. 2000. [Unnecessary operations in the exercise of surgery. A topic of our times with serious implications in medical ethics]. *Gac Med Mex* 136 (2):183-8.

239. Rutkow, I. M. 1987. Surgical operations in the United States: 1979 to 1984. *Surgery* 101 (2):192-200.

240. Rutkow, I. M. 1997. Surgical operations in the United States. Then (1983) and now (1994). *Arch Surg* 132 (9):983-90.

241. Linnemann, M. U., and H. H. Bulow. 1993. [Infections after insertion of epidural catheters]. *Ugeskr Laeger* 155 (30):2350-2.

242. Seres, J. L., and R. I. Newman. 1989. Perspectives on surgical indications. Implications for controls. *Clin J Pain* 5 (2):131-6.

243. Chassin, M. R., J. Kosecoff, R. E. Park, C. M. Winslow, K. L. Kahn, N. J. Merrick, J. Keesey, A. Fink, D. H. Solomon, and R. H. Brook. 1987. Does inappropriate use explain geographic variations in the use of health care services? A study of three procedures. *JAMA* 258 (18):2533-7.

244. Available at: http://www.ahrq.gov/data/ hcup/ hcupnet.htm. (accessed May 22, 2006).

245. Leape LL. Unnecessary surgery. Health Serv Res. 1989 Aug;24(3):351-407.

246. Available at: http://www.ahrq.gov/data/ hcup/ hcupnet.htm. (accessed May 22, 2006).

247. Lazarou, J., B. H. Pomeranz, and P. N. Corey. 1998. Incidence of adverse drug reactions in hospitalized patients: a meta-analysis of prospective studies. *JAMA* 279 (15):1200-5.

248. Innovations Exchange: Checklist-Plus-Technology System . . . , Enhances Required Preoperative Process Compliance, AHRQ, September 29, 2008. http://www.innovations.ahrq.gov/content. aspx?id=2262 (accessed February 1, 2009).

249. Ibid.

250. Houts, Marshall. *Where Death Delights*. (New York: Coward McCann, 1967), pp. 253-254.

251. InjuryBoard.com. Virginia Has Special Medical Malpractice Law on Retained Surgical Towels, *January 22, 2009*. http://norfolk.injuryboard. com/medical-malpractice/virginia-has-special-medical-malpractice-law-on-retained-surgical-towels.aspx?googleid=255786 (accessed February 1, 2009).

252. Ibid.

253. Stark, K. and J. Goldstein, When surgical instruments are left behind - in patients: In the Phila. area, about 80 mistakes are made a year, *Philadelphia Inquirer*, February 1, 2004; reprinted by Committee for Justice for All. http://www.saynotocaps.org/newsarticles/ When%20surgical%20instruments%20are%20 left%20behind%20-%20in%20patients.htm (accessed February 1, 2009).

254. InjuryBoard.com. Hospitals are Still Neglecting to Report Serious Mistakes—Are Medical Malpractice Lawsuits the Public's Only Hope? *InjuryBoard.com, January 30, 2009*. http://cherryhill. injuryboard.com/medical-malpractice/hospitals-are-still-neglecting-to-report-serious-mistakes-are-medical-malpractice-lawsuits-the-publics-only-hope.aspx?googleid=256380 *(accessed February 1, 2009)*.

255. Haynes, A. B., M.D., M.P.H., (Harvard School of Public Health, Massachusetts General Hospital), et al., A Surgical Safety Checklist to Reduce Morbidity and Mortality in a Global Population, *New England Journal of Medicine* 360(5): 491-499,

January 29, 2009. http://content.nejm.org/cgi/content/full/NEJMsa0810119 (accessed February 1, 2009).

256. Nagourney, E, Checklist Reduces Deaths in Surgery, *New York Times,* January 14, 2009. http://www.nytimes.com/2009/01/20/health/20surgery.html (accessed February 1, 2009).

257. Ibid.

258. Office of Technology Assessment, US Congress. Assessing the Efficacy and Safety of Medical Technologies. Washington DC: Office of Technology Assessment, US Congress; 1978.

259. Available at: www.wws.princeton.edu/ota/disk1/1995/9562_n.html. (accessed May 22, 2006).

260. US Office of Technology Assessment. OTA Archive, August 1996. http://www.access.gpo.gov/ota/ (accessed February 1, 2009).

261. InjuryBoard.com. Hospitals are Still Neglecting to Report Serious Mistakes - Are Medical Malpractice Lawsuits the Public's Only Hope? InjuryBoard.com, January 30, 2009. http://cherryhill.injuryboard.com/medical-malpractice/hospitals-are-still-neglecting-to-report-serious-mistakes-are-medical-malpractice-lawsuits-the-publics-only-hope.aspx?googleid=256380 (accessed February 1, 2009).

262. Ibid.

263. Ibid.

264. Zhan, C., and M. R. Miller. 2003. Excess length of stay, charges, and mortality attributable to

medical injuries during hospitalization. *JAMA* 290 (14):1868-74.

265. Available at: http://www.ahrq.gov/news/ ress/ pr2003/injurypr.htm. (Accessed May 22, 2006).

266. Weingart, S. N., and L. I. Iezzoni. 2003. Looking for medical injuries where the light is bright. *JAMA* 290 (14):1917-9.

267. Macmahon, B. 1962. Prenatal x-ray exposure and childhood cancer. *J Natl Cancer Inst* 28:1173-91.

268. Available at: http://hps.org/publicinformation/ ate/q1084.html. (accessed May 22, 2006).

269. Gofman, J.W. Radiation from Medical Procedures in the Pathogenesis of Cancer and Ischemic Heart Disease: Dose-Response Studies with Physicians per 100,000 Population. (San Francisco, CA: CNR Books, 1999).

270. Gofman, J.W. Preventing Breast Cancer: The Story of a Major, Proven, Preventable Cause of This Disease, 2nd ed. (San Francisco, CA: CNR Books, 1996).

271. Twomly, R. "Full-Body Ct Screening: Preventing or Producing Cancer?" J Natl Cancer Inst96, no. 22 (2004): 1650-1.

272. Ibid.

273. Ibid.

274. Sarno, J.E. Healing Back Pain: The Mind-Body Connection. Warner Books; 1991.

275. http://www.ahrq.gov/data/ hcup/hcupnet.htm. (accessed May 22, 2006).

276. Siu, A. L., F. A. Sonnenberg, W. G. Manning, G. A. Goldberg, E. S. Bloomfield, J. P. Newhouse, and R. H. Brook. 1986. Inappropriate use of hospitals in a randomized trial of health insurance plans. *N Engl J Med* 315 (20):1259-66.

277. Siu, A. L., W. G. Manning, and B. Benjamin. 1990. Patient, provider and hospital characteristics associated with inappropriate hospitalization. *Am J Public Health* 80 (10):1253-6.

278. Eriksen, B. O., I. S. Kristiansen, E. Nord, J. F. Pape, S. M. Almdahl, A. Hensrud, and S. Jaeger. 1999. The cost of inappropriate admissions: a study of health benefits and resource utilization in a department of internal medicine. *J Intern Med* 246 (4):379-87.

279. Siu, A. L., F. A. Sonnenberg, W. G. Manning, G. A. Goldberg, E. S. Bloomfield, J. P. Newhouse, and R. H. Brook. 1986. Inappropriate use of hospitals in a randomized trial of health insurance plans. *N Engl J Med* 315 (20):1259-66.

280. Siu, A. L., W. G. Manning, and B. Benjamin. 1990. Patient, provider and hospital characteristics associated with inappropriate hospitalization. *Am J Public Health* 80 (10):1253-6.

281. Eriksen, B. O., I. S. Kristiansen, E. Nord, J. F. Pape, S. M. Almdahl, A. Hensrud, and S. Jaeger. 1999. The cost of inappropriate admissions: a study of health benefits and resource utilization in a department of internal medicine. *J Intern Med* 246 (4):379-87.

282. Available at: http://www.ahrq.gov/data/ hcup/ hcupnet.htm. (accessed May 22, 2006).

283. http://www.ahrq.gov/data/ hcup/hcupnet.htm. (accessed May 22, 2006).

284. Siu, A. L., F. A. Sonnenberg, W. G. Manning, G. A. Goldberg, E. S. Bloomfield, J. P. Newhouse, and R. H. Brook. 1986. Inappropriate use of hospitals in a randomized trial of health insurance plans. *N Engl J Med* 315 (20):1259-66.

285. Siu, A. L., W. G. Manning, and B. Benjamin. 1990. Patient, provider and hospital characteristics associated with inappropriate hospitalization. *Am J Public Health* 80 (10):1253-6.

286. Eriksen, B. O., I. S. Kristiansen, E. Nord, J. F. Pape, S. M. Almdahl, A. Hensrud, and S. Jaeger. 1999. The cost of inappropriate admissions: a study of health benefits and resource utilization in a department of internal medicine. *J Intern Med* 246 (4):379-87.

287. Weinstein, R. A. 1998. Nosocomial infection update. *Emerg Infect Dis* 4 (3):416-20.

288. Fourth Decennial International Conference on Nosocomial and Healthcare-Associated Infections. Morbidity and Mortality Weekly Report. February 25, 2000, Vol. 49, No. 7, p. 138.

289. HealthGrades Quality Study: Patient Safety in American Hospitals, April 2004.

290. Pittet, D., A. Simon, S. Hugonnet, C. L. Pessoa-Silva, V. Sauvan, and T. V. Perneger. 2004. Hand hygiene among physicians: performance, beliefs, and perceptions. *Ann Intern Med* 141 (1):1-8.

291. HealthGrades Quality Study: Second Annual Patient Safety in American Hospitals, May 2005.

292. Starfield, B. 2000. Is US health really the best in the world? *JAMA* 284 (4):483-5.

293. Starfield, B. 2000. Deficiencies in US medical care. *JAMA* 284 (17):2184-5.

294. Weingart, S. N., L. Wilson R. Mc, R. W. Gibberd, and B. Harrison. 2000. Epidemiology of medical error. *West J Med* 172 (6):390-3.

295. Showalter, E. Hystories: *Hysterical Epidemics and Modern Media*. (New York: Columbia University Press, 1997).

296. Available at: http://college.hmco.com/history/readerscomp/women/html/wh_001200_alternativeh.htm. (accessed May 16, 2006).

297. Thacker, S.B., D. Stroup, M. Chang. Continuous electronic heart rate monitoring for fetal assessment during labor (Cochrane Review). In: The Cochrane Library, issue 1, 2003. Oxford: Update Software.

298. Cole, C. 2003. Admission electronic fetal monitoring does not improve neonatal outcomes. *J Fam Pract* 52 (6):443-4.

299. Nelson, H. D., L. L. Humphrey, P. Nygren, S. M. Teutsch, and J. D. Allan. 2002. Postmenopausal hormone replacement therapy: scientific review. *JAMA* 288 (7):872-81.

300. Nelson, H. D. 2002. Assessing benefits and harms of hormone replacement therapy: clinical applications. *JAMA* 288 (7):882-4.

301. Fletcher, S. W., and G. A. Colditz. 2002. Failure of estrogen plus progestin therapy for prevention. *JAMA* 288 (3):366-8.

302. Rossouw, J. E., G. L. Anderson, R. L. Prentice, A. Z. LaCroix, C. Kooperberg, M. L. Stefanick, R. D. Jackson, S. A. Beresford, B. V. Howard, K. C. Johnson, J. M. Kotchen, and J. Ockene. 2002. Risks and benefits of estrogen plus progestin in healthy postmenopausal women: principal results From the Women's Health Initiative randomized controlled trial. *JAMA* 288 (3):321-33.

303. Hysterectomy prevalence and death rates for cervical cancer—United States, 1965-1988. 1992. *MMWR Morb Mortal Wkly Rep* 41 (2):17-20. http://www.cdc.gov/mmwr/preview/mmwrhtml/00015908.htm (accessed February 1, 2009).

304. Rutkow, I. M. 1986. Obstetric and gynecologic operations in the United States, 1979 to 1984. *Obstet Gynecol* 67 (6):755-9.

305. Family Practice News. February 15, 1995:29.

306. Sakala, C. 1993. Medically unnecessary cesarean section births: introduction to a symposium. *Soc Sci Med* 37 (10):1177-98.

307. VanHam, M.A., P.W. van Dongen, J. Mulder. Maternal consequences of cesarean section. A retrospective study of intraoperative and postoperative maternal complications of cesarean section during a 10-year period. Eur J Obstet Reprod Biol. 1997 Jul;74(1):1-6.

308. Xakellis, G. C., R. Frantz, and A. Lewis. 1995. Cost of pressure ulcer prevention in long-term care. *J Am Geriatr Soc* 43 (5):496-501.

309. Barczak, C. A., R. I. Barnett, E. J. Childs, and L. M. Bosley. 1997. Fourth national pressure ulcer prevalence survey. *Adv Wound Care* 10 (4):18-26.

310. Available at: http://www.injuryboard.com/ view. cfm/Article=3005 (accessed May 22, 2006).

311. Available at: http://www.cmwf.org/programs/ elders/burger_mal_386.asp. (accessed May 22, 2006).

312. Barczak, C. A., R. I. Barnett, E. J. Childs, and L. M. Bosley. 1997. Fourth national pressure ulcer prevalence survey. *Adv Wound Care* 10 (4):18-26.

313. Kotulak, R. Doctors' haste seen hurting patient: study says the push for quick treatment detracts from care. *Chicago Tribune online edition*, 10 May 2005. http://www.chicagotribune.com/features/ health/ (no longer available here); available at Committee for Justice for All: Patient Safety and Doctor Discipline, CJA President Attorney Peter I. Fallk, Dr. Persell quote is on website. http://www. saynotocaps.org/patientsafety.shtml (accessed January 28, 2009).

314. Available at: http://www.cmwf.org/programs/ elders/burger_mal_386.asp. (accessed May 22, 2006).

315. Available at: http://www.house.gov/waxman (accessed May 22, 2006).

316. Mitka, M. 1998. Unacceptable nursing home deaths unautopsied. *JAMA* 280 (12):1038-9.

317. Medical Review of North Carolina, Inc. New data is in on North Carolina's nursing home residents. July 21, 2003.

318. Weinstein, R. A. 1998. Nosocomial infection update. *Emerg Infect Dis* 4 (3):416-20.

319. Available at: http://www.house.gov/waxman (accessed May 22, 2006).

320. Available at: http://www.house.gov/waxman (accessed May 22, 2006).

321. Centers for Medicare & Medicaid Services. Report to Congress: Appropriateness of Minimum Nurse Staffing Ratios in Nursing Homes: Phase II Final Report. December 24, 2001.

322. National Citizens' Coalition for Nursing Home Reform. Consumer group criticizes Thompson letter dismissing report on dangerous staffing levels in nursing homes [news release]. Washington, DC: March 22, 2002.

323. Bergstrom, N., B. Braden, M. Kemp, M. Champagne, and E. Ruby. 1996. Multi-site study of incidence of pressure ulcers and the relationship between risk level, demographic characteristics, diagnoses, and prescription of preventive interventions. *J Am Geriatr Soc* 44 (1):22-30.

324. Miles, S. H. 2002. Concealing accidental nursing home deaths. *HEC Forum* 14 (3):224-34.

325. Corey, T. S., B. Weakley-Jones, G. R. Nichols, 2nd, and H. H. Theuer. 1992. Unnatural deaths in nursing home patients. *J Forensic Sci* 37 (1):222-7.

326. Lloyd-Jones, D. M., D. O. Martin, M. G. Larson, and D. Levy. 1998. Accuracy of death certificates for coding coronary heart disease as the cause of death. *Ann Intern Med* 129 (12):1020-6.

327. Thomas, D. R., C. D. Zdrowski, M. M. Wilson, K. C. Conright, C. Lewis, S. Tariq, and J. E. Morley. 2002. Malnutrition in subacute care. *Am J Clin Nutr* 75 (2):308-13.

328. Robinson, B. E. 1995. Death by destruction of will. Lest we forget. *Arch Intern Med* 155 (20):2250-1.

329. Capezuti, E., N. E. Strumpf, L. K. Evans, J. A. Grisso, and G. Maislin. 1998. The relationship between physical restraint removal and falls and injuries among nursing home residents. *J Gerontol A Biol Sci Med Sci* 53 (1):M47-52.

330. Phillips, C. D., C. Hawes, and B. E. Fries. 1993. Reducing the use of physical restraints in nursing homes: will it increase costs? *Am J Public Health* 83 (3):342-8.

331. Miles, S. H., and P. Irvine. 1992. Deaths caused by physical restraints. *Gerontologist* 32 (6):762-6.

332. Annas, G. J. 1999. The last resort—the use of physical restraints in medical emergencies. *N Engl J Med* 341 (18):1408-12.

333. Parker, K., and S. H. Miles. 1997. Deaths caused by bedrails. *J Am Geriatr Soc* 45 (7):797-802.

334. Katz, P. R., and G. Seidel. 1990. Nursing home autopsies. Survey of physician attitudes and practice patterns. *Arch Pathol Lab Med* 114 (2):145-7.

335. Reuters Health. Overmedication of US seniors. May 21, 2003.

336. Drug Benefit Trends. Average number of prescriptions by HMOs increases. 2002 Sep 12;14(8).

337. Drug Benefit Trends. Average number of prescriptions by HMOs increases. 2002 Sep 12;14(8).

338. Kaiser Family Foundation. Prescription Drug Trends. November, 2001.

339. Williams, B. R., M. B. Nichol, B. Lowe, P. S. Yoon, J. S. McCombs, and J. Margolies. 1999. Medication use in residential care facilities for the elderly. *Ann Pharmacother* 33 (2):149-55.

340. Available at: http://www.aarp.org/prescription-drugs (accessed May 22, 2006).

341. Office of the Attorney General, Department of Justice, State of California. California reaches $100 million multi-state settlement with drug giant Mylan over alleged price-fixing scheme [press release]. Sacramento, CA; July 12, 2000.

342. Available at: http://www.wral.com/money/2026364/detail.html (accessed May 22, 2006).

343. Available at: www.education.guardian.co.uk/businessofresearch/comment/ 0,9976,606260,00.html (accessed May 22, 2006).

344. Available at: http://www.aarp.org/Articles/a2003-03-07-supplements.html (accessed May 22, 2006).

345. Bernabei, R., G. Gambassi, K. Lapane, F. Landi, C. Gatsonis, R. Dunlop, L. Lipsitz, K. Steel, and V. Mor. 1998. Management of pain in elderly patients with cancer. SAGE Study Group. Systematic Assessment of Geriatric Drug Use via Epidemiology. *JAMA* 279 (23):1877-82.

346. Abel, U. 1992. Chemotherapy of advanced epithelial cancer—a critical review. *Biomed Pharmacother* 46 (10):439-52.

347. World Health Organization. Press Release Bulletin #9. December 17, 2001.

348. Angell, M. 2000. Is academic medicine for sale? *N Engl J Med* 342 (20):1516-8.

349. McKenzie, J. Conflict of interest? Medical journal changes policy of finding independent doctors [transcript]. *ABC News*. June 12, 2002.

350. Crossen C. *Tainted Truth: The Manipulation of Fact in America*. (New York: Simon & Schuster; 1994).

351. Mundy A. Pressured, Schools Review Ties to Drug Firms, *Wall Street Journal*, September 11, 2008. http://online.wsj.com/article/SB122109019382321441.html (accessed January 28, 2009).

352. Jalloh, A. C.U. Supports Disclosure of Univ. Research, *The Cornell Daily Sun*, October 7, 2008. http://cornellsun.com/section/news/content/2008/10/07/cu-supports-disclosure-univ-research-funding (accessed January 28, 2009).

353. Medical News Today. Grassley, Kohl Say Public Should Know When Pharmaceutical Makers Give Money To Doctors, USA, September 8, 2007. http://www.medicalnewstoday.com/articles/81822.php (accessed January 28, 2009).

354. Weiner, J. Smoking and cancer: the cigarette papers: how the industry is trying to smoke us all. *The Nation*. January 1, 1996:11-18.

355. Available at: www.tobacco.org/resources/history/ tobacco_history.html (acccessed May 22, 2006).

356. Associated Press. Panel names estrogen as carcinogen. *The Washington Post*. December 16, 2000:A05.

357. Cole, C. 2003. Admission electronic fetal monitoring does not improve neonatal outcomes. *J Fam Pract* 52 (6):443-4.

358. MSNBC staff and wire reports. Estrogen hikes ovarian cancer risk. July 16, 2002. Grady D. Study recommends NOT using hormone therapy for bone loss. *New York Times*. October 1, 2003.

359. Anderson, G. L., H. L. Judd, A. M. Kaunitz, D. H. Barad, S. A. Beresford, M. Pettinger, J. Liu, S. G. McNeeley, and A. M. Lopez. 2003. Effects of estrogen plus progestin on gynecologic cancers and associated diagnostic procedures: the Women's Health Initiative randomized trial. *JAMA* 290 (13):1739-48.

360. Chlebowski, R. T., S. L. Hendrix, R. D. Langer, M. L. Stefanick, M. Gass, D. Lane, R. J. Rodabough, M. A. Gilligan, M. G. Cyr, C. A. Thomson, J. Khandekar, H. Petrovitch, and A. McTiernan. 2003. Influence of estrogen plus progestin on breast cancer and mammography in healthy postmenopausal women: the Women's Health Initiative Randomized Trial. *JAMA* 289 (24):3243-53.

361. Wassertheil-Smoller, S., S. L. Hendrix, M. Limacher, G. Heiss, C. Kooperberg, A. Baird, T. Kotchen, J. D. Curb, H. Black, J. E. Rossouw, A. Aragaki, M. Safford, E. Stein, S. Laowattana, and

W. J. Mysiw. 2003. Effect of estrogen plus pro-gestin on stroke in postmenopausal women: the Women's Health Initiative: a randomized trial. *JAMA* 289 (20):2673-84.

362. Shumaker, S. A., C. Legault, S. R. Rapp, L. Thal, R. B. Wallace, J. K. Ockene, S. L. Hendrix, B. N. Jones, 3rd, A. R. Assaf, R. D. Jackson, J. M. Kotchen, S. Wassertheil-Smoller, and J. Wac-tawski-Wende. 2003. Estrogen plus progestin and the incidence of dementia and mild cogni-tive impairment in postmenopausal women: the Women's Health Initiative Memory Study: a randomized controlled trial. *JAMA* 289 (20):2651-62.

363. Beral, V. 2003. Breast cancer and hormone-replacement therapy in the Million Women Study. *Lancet* 362 (9382):419-27.

364. Nainggolan, L and C.Vega, MD. Breast Cancer Risk Remains After Stopping HRT, (based on the source Heiss, G., Wallace, R., Anderson, G.L., et al. Health risks and benefits 3 years after stop-ping randomized treatment with estrogen and progestin. *JAMA*. 2008;299:1036-1045), *Med-scape Medical News*, March 5, 2008; http://www.medscape.com/viewarticle/571032 (accessed February 1, 2009).

Index

G

H